Dopamine Detox

How Dopamine Detox Can Help You Take Control of Your Life

(Get Your Brain to Remove Distractions and Focus to Turn Hard Things Into Base Instincts)

Gregory Clark

Published By **Ryan Princeton**

Gregory Clark

Dopamine Detox: How Dopamine Detox Can Help You Take Control of Your Life (Get Your Brain to Remove Distractions and Focus to Turn Hard Things Into Base Instincts)

ISBN 978-1-998038-59-6

Legal & Disclaimer

Table Of Contents

Chapter 1: Motivated By Dopamine

Human beings embody life force that was designed to be masters of their own fate and take control of their lives. Just like fish with breathing gills that allow them to breathe underwater, or even birds equipped with wings that allow them to fly in over the sky in all directions, we are perfectly suited to adapt to the environment, but to master the environment. But, despite the fact that we're the perfect species made to conquer the world regardless of the challenges that life presents, a lot people aren't performing to the fullest of our potential.

The world is tossed about like dead leaves in a turbulent whirlwind. Rubber balls are tossed around in the ocean's waves. It is easy to accept jobs that aren't in alignment with our God-given goal because we feel stifled by our family, society and our friends. Insecure and inadequate, we feel and consequently cover ourselves in masks in order to hide the underlying fears. The masks we wear can be described as material wealth, wealth or positions of power, accomplishments in work or other jobs, etc. They aren't undesirable in and of themselves However, a lot of people chase in search of these things so that they can cover up their true identity and to bolster their self-esteem against the perceived lack of self-confidence.

The main reason that we go in ego-driven trips is because of the fact we're not connected to the inner self. Our bodies are always removed from our source of strength. The apparent disconnect causes a void that requires to be filled.

It is easy to be unhappy with the circumstances and frequently are unable to act and alter the course of events. We all feel that we need to fill in the gap and re-energise our own thoughts and contemplate the meaning of life. We put our personalities and our ego in front of their mirrors of heart and ask ourselves deep-seated questions. In all certainty, when we think about these questions of soul searching and the answer is always right in front of at us with a stern stare. A quiet voice whispers to us during those times in silence and contemplation. We immediately know what to do when we are able to pay attention.

We seek satisfaction in various ways. Our desire to avoid suffering is a part of all of us. Anything that brings our hearts joy or happiness such as the altruistic act making up a fraudulent scheme or even murdering someone and the ultimate aim of all our efforts is enjoyment. All of us are pleasure-seeking creatures. It is a pleasure that has received various names, donned in

3

different clothes and served to us in different ways. Many call it destiny, people mistake it with material items. Many seek its presence by way of religion. A few are seeking to have it by force. Some seek it through getting married, starting a family or even focusing on their the career.

The issue is that we aren't listening to the voice, but we always hear. The voice of reason rationality, consciousness, or spirit will always be there to guide us to stay on the right track or are not aligned with the goals we set. The issue is hearing. The majority of the time, we aren't taking the less traveled path. We tend to ignore our inner voice that questions our motivations, motives and objectives. We are reluctant to go in the flame to get the pleasure we seek. We look for less stressful methods to enjoy that feeling. We look for ways to get around drinking, drugs, video games, binge-film watching, etc. We indulge in escapism searching for that everlasting 'high to lift our spirits from the lowest points in our lives.

Escapism's biggest drawback is that it's an uncontrollable beast that has to constantly fed. Escapism is a way to escape the reality of life into a dreamlike state. The place we block away from the reality around us by removing its frequency and turn off. We don't want to confront our anxieties and problems and put ourselves in the flames that will melt the flaws in us and make ourselves as flawless as a pearl. We keep our minds off uncomfortable situations that arise within our daily lives, constantly trying to get the pleasure from escape.

It's not a long-term solution because reality always sets the scene. Rent for living in a paradise for fools will always be paid via an actual check (or check). Escapism is similar to an fog, and the rush from the reality of things is sure to dispel it. The moment that the intensity of the high fades it is time to fall from our dream state, we're leaving naked and bare as we stand before the judge of our conscience and decision of our lives. We do not sit to be convicted. It's time to escape from the pressures of daily life. Therefore, we end up engaging in activities which distract us from our petty problems.

One of the essential instruments that has been left to us in order to help us navigate through life's challenges includes the brain. The brain of a human is an amazing tool but it is it is also an interesting thing. Sometimes, it cooperates and helps us complete tasks. However, most of the time it's non-cooperative and causes us to put off and become stuck. This is a dual-edged weapon and it works however you use it. Knowing our emotions and brain is the key ingredient to success and a balanced life.

There are numerous chemicals stored within the brain, which enable us to express emotions through our body speech. These feelings are caused through chemicals that can either encourage us to do things or cool the flames of our soul and can cause us to be discouraged. The chemicals that trigger these emotions are sent out via neurotransmitters. They permit impulses to pass between cells through the nerve system. Neurotransmitters allow us to experience pleasure or hurt, movements of muscles, as well as the emotional reaction to the stimulus.

The neurotransmitter used to connect our brains to emotions is dopamine. It's sometimes described as the molecule that gives us more. Dopamine plays a role in the reward system of the brain since it induces feelings of joy and drives our need. Dopamine levels in the brain increase as we engage in activities that give us pleasure as well as pleasure. In other words, when we're smitten, driven by passion or relationship, the level of dopamine rises in response to the idea of someone or the prospect of being with them or spend time with them. When we anticipate something that is desirable for example, food, money or promotion and a new vehicle, an upgrade to our home, the coming of a child or something 'good' happening in our lives and our levels of dopamine increase.

Similar to when we engage with escapist activities like drinking, drugs and gambling our levels of dopamine go up. The reason for this is that the brain releases dopamine when it is responding to satisfaction or fulfillment and activates the pleasure cells of the brain. This increases the excitement the pulse increases and we are eagerly anticipating what we might be able to. It's like looking forward to meeting your new lover, or the score of a game or the exam results.

Dopamine feeds off the thrill of novelty of our future-oriented hopes as well as our hopes and dreams. It is the embodiment of our ideals as well as our dreams. We have hopes and desires. The most brilliant work or extraordinary feat could be completed without a burst of dopamine. Every brilliant act, whether good or not, could be accomplished without an injection of dopamine.

Every activity that relies by reward or pleasure is powered by dopamine. The reason we get obsessed on certain subjects and drop fascination with others is due to the way that our brain interprets these events and releases dopamine according to. If we participate in an activity that causes an increase in dopamine levels, it is likely that we will repeat the same action.

You might be tired frequently, or feel tired throughout the day. It is difficult to find motivation, you feel overwhelmed, are suffering from depression or feel overloaded by the demands in your daily life. You are irritable and put off work often. Your energy is low or perhaps you're dealing with an addiction which you cannot beat. There is something that you believe is taking over your life. It's not your passion, enthusiasm or you feel depressed moving through the day with no guidance. It's possible that your brain has run out of dopamine.

Chapter 2: An Molecule Of Pleasure Or Novelty?

Medical scientists and psychologists studying addiction performed a large portion of the earlier research in the field of dopamine. The 1930s were a time when the study of addictive behavior was an emerging field it was believed that addicts were morally sloppy or lacking the willpower.

It wasn't until the groundbreaking research that was made by Professor. Arvid Carlsson, a Swedish neuroscientist who discovered the connection between dopamine and motivation in relation to addiction was identified. Before his study the majority of scientists held believing that dopamine is only a signpost for the presence of noradrenaline (Norepinephrine) which is an important brain hormone to regulate the heart rate, as well as mobilizing the brain and body for the execution of. Dopamine was thought to be a substance that is connected to motor sensors as well as physical movements.

But, the findings from studies conducted by Carlsson's on rabbits proved that, if the dopamine levels in the brain were inadequate, the neural pathways that the brain regulates the body's movement could not work properly.

Carlsson found that cutting down on dopamine levels of rabbits made their bodies inactive, showing symptoms that were similar symptoms similar to those experienced by Parkinson's patients. The discovery of his later led to the way to research to find treatment strategies for patients suffering from Parkinson's disease. This research then led to addiction studies.

The 1980s saw Wolfram Schultz was the German neuroscientist, improved the direction of his research following several experiments with rats. The results of his research showed dopamine's involvement in the reward system in the brain. To verify their theories, Schultz and his team put apple pieces in front of screens and observed dopamine activity in a rats' brains as they dined in the food. The researchers found that in the excitement of food Dopamine levels within the brain of a rat increased. Schultz discovered that anytime you are anticipating an outcome, there's likely to be an upsurge in dopamine production in the brain.

Another study (conducted using human subjects) A team of researchers sought to study the effect of dopamine to the brain of humans. Scientists monitored the brain activity of the brain of participants after they were given doses of cocaine. In the course of the study, subjects were asked to rate their level of euphoria experienced at different points. The researchers found that the activity of dopamine was directly related to the degree of happiness. It is therefore clear that the greater dopamine levels more intense the feeling of emotion of the euphoria. When the levels of dopamine decreased, as is the sensation of euphoria.

Although it's easy to think that dopamine can be the catalyst behind our desire to do something in response to perceived benefits, some caution must be used here since such beliefs are bogus. Human desires, as they say are endless. That is exactly how we function. of dopamine. When we achieve what we are looking for Do we feel that we are empty time? Then we ask ourselves why it was that initially which prompted us to invest an enormous amount of time and effort in search for these goals? It is like the true seeker who is at the top of their mountain, only to realize that the summit is actually an esplanade with mountain ranges to conquer. The quotation from J.P. Morgan aptly encapsulates the downward slope of dopamine to the extent that your eyes will allow, at the point you reach and look around, you'll see even more.

Dopamine being referred to as a "pleasure molecule" that is a driver of motivation and desire is not sufficient, because studies have revealed that the functioning of this brain chemical are far more complicated than we had previously believed. In a study that was jointly that was conducted by a group comprising psychologists at North Kentucky University and Washington University the use of food was employed to measure dopamine levels in rats. Food containers were placed in a rats cage to see how dopamine levels changed in response to anticipation of and the consumption from food. The results showed that there was an increase in dopamine levels within the brain of rats when food is dropped into their cage. But, once this action began to become routineized, the scientists observed that, even though the rats took in the food with as much enthusiasm as they had the initial time, the levels of dopamine decreased.

Dopamine is a chemical that only is elevated or increases whenever there is an expectation of new reward. The reward is not a feeling of satisfaction - which is the ultimate goal - it's the chemical that creates excitement, or the anticipation of the possibility of a fresh or exciting feeling. Simply put, only unanticipated results stimulate dopamine.

It's because of this neurotransmitter, which always causes us to want more. However, once you have what we wanted or were enthralled with, the brain's neurotransmitter switches off, removing any sensations of happiness we experienced initially which makes us feel empty and unfulfilling. We are left in a state of craving the pleasure. So, we engage into these cravings over and over to try and get back to our euphoria which leads us into the cycle of addiction.

It can also be extrapolated and incorporated into our daily life and our relationships. Once we have met the person who we have always wanted or aspired on, we're overwhelmed. Sometime we get too in love with the person that we are able to eat or rest. After we and have settled into our relationship, we discover that the attractive qualities that we used to admire in our partner have disappeared. It's been a while since we felt the desire to be like a candle blowing in the breeze. The excitement wears off, and we begin to get familiar with the individual. We become comfortable and relaxed because the thrill of being a part of that person in the first place has waned. Maybe this is the reason it is said that being absent makes hearts grow more affectionate. The reason was that the brain stops releases dopamine in response to the thoughts of the individual since that enjoyable experience is now complete.

An excellent example is seen in the world of sex (which is something that a large number men can identify with!). In the world of sexual intimacy, lots of males are high on dopamine (and ladies, too but don't get it wrong!). Men go out in search of a female to get her number, and then decides to bring her home. In a flash the guy loses interest in the woman. Also, if a woman is approached by an individual who resembles her but later finds out that (s)he does not seem to be what she imagined after having a few minutes with him. The reason for this is that the dopamine in their system has worn off and they feel less interested in their connection.

Studies have revealed that the majority of unions end up breaking up two to five years following. It is due to the honeymoon stage that is fueled by dopamine is over. The desire to live your entire life together is now replaced by boringness, monotony and a sense of familiarity. No more thrills or excitement because the dopamine which fueled those assumed love feeling have drained away.

Filmmakers, advertisers as well as business owners have consciously or not, have come up with ways to boost our dopamine levels. They first provide a sneak peek of the film, which allows the audience to see a preview of what we can expect or take pre-orders for new items that will come out in just three months. This is all geared towards boost your dopamine levels to ensure that, when the item is released, you are eager to get the item. A few months later and you are left wondering what prompted you to purchase the item at all and discover that the film was hyped up. The suspense of films that keep viewers glued in anticipation of what will happen to your favourite character is powered by dopamine. This is exactly what hyping is all about. It increases the levels of dopamine because you are expecting an outcome!

You might have wanted something awful, such as an online game, brand new car, a bigger shoe, or a new house to explore the world, or travel to the place you've always wanted to visit. Dopamine fuels your anticipation to get the item. Once you have these items in the course of time it is when the excitement or pleasure that comes with the pursuit wears off. The duration of time that dopamine disappears varies dependent on the amount or amount of dopamine that the brain releases in pursuit of the desired goal. It could take hours, days or even years for it to disappear, and happens eventually. After this it leaves us feeling empty and depleted. Then we begin looking to find something else that could bring us the same satisfaction of anxiety, excitement, and a desire for pleasure which we had built up prior to the time reaching our objectives. Dopamine is a term used to describe a pit that never ends, as well as an unending desire, a tidal wave of desire that never stops seeking more and sucking us into the trough, but never leaving our hearts content. Because nature hates vacuums in which to fill, the absence of this satisfaction must be filled again and repeatedly. It can lead to addictions since we operate in a state that is over our norm.

It can happen when getting the chance to raise your salary or get promoted. Funny thing is that as humans, we are addicted to dopamine. We are awestruck by new experiences like new adventures, challenges and the excitement of having an infant, or even falling in with love. We are addicted to adrenaline to a certain extent. Once our hopes become what we get and we get it, the levels of dopamine drop. Do we really believe that we will be chasing things, having unending desires and needs that go unnoticed when we acquire the items? It's not so. If we are looking to gain satisfaction from what are available, it's vital that we remove our brains from the dopamine.

Chapter 3: Dopamine Triggers

Dopamine itself isn't bad. It can be extremely beneficial to people because it allows us to put off gratification, which allows us to work towards the objectives, goals and goals we've set for us. The problem with many people is that they engage in an abundance of actions we engage in which have a high level of dopamine which could be detrimental to our health. A few of these activities can be considered conscious, while the vast majority of them happen unconsciously.

Dopamine can be great in small amounts, because it lets us take pleasure in food, appreciate moments, and cherish connections. If we do push the dopamine pathway far enough, it can lead to addiction. A few of the different ways that dopamine can be triggered within our brains are listed in the following.

Foods high in sugar

Humans are normal to want sweeter foods rather than bitter, even though they can be good for the health of our bodies and overall well-being. Yet, the desire to eat sweet foods could be just as powerful as substances such as heroin and cocaine. When a person ingests sugar, the brain releases massive surges of dopamine that are like how it responds to the consumption of heroin and cocaine. Since the brain perceives sweet foods as beneficial for the body (or the taste buds) that is why it releases massive levels of dopamine prior to the start of the consumption. Researchers have been able to speculate that this may result from our bodies have evolved to search for things that are rich in calories with long periods of.

When you eat cookies, junk food doughnut, cookie, or any other it is, your body responds to dopamine. It is the reason you feel that desire for sweets. Imagine it, experience it and, if you've got it, you'll feel less appealing after just a few bites. After the fourth or fifth bite it's time to consider which reason you bought the cupcake that you decided not to purchase initially. However, you continue to eat it when you make a new resolution that results in an addiction to sweets or binge eating.

It is also recognized as being intense during the beginning stages of recovery for addicts and alcoholics. Drinking alcohol contains a significant level of sugar. Therefore, an alcohol-related body as well as the brain are accustomed to the highest levels of sugar due to regularly or frequently drinking. The results of studies have revealed that as a result of the reduction of dopamine that is triggered by alcohol and drugs and other stimuli, our brains crave alternatives sweet foods that will always have the same impact. After a person is sober, their brains are stripped from the high in sugar that it's familiar with from drinking alcohol drinks. The result is a greater craving for sweet gobbles. This is the reason why lots of alcohol drinkers tend to enjoy the pleasures of sweets and candy in this transition period.

Pornography/Masturbation

Since the past few years, neuroscientific research has revealed the connection between the reward system in the brain and sexuality in humans, casting fresh light on unhealthy and problematic sexual behaviors. Doctor. Valerie Voon, neuropsychiatrist at Cambridge University discovered that the men's brains are known to show structure changes that are in the same region that drug addicts do. As the majority of these examples were illustrated using sexual activities, this segment would be about sexually unhealthy behaviour and the stimulant that is associated with of masturbation as well as pornography.

Pornography is driven 200% by dopamine. And the porn industry has devised strategies to keep their audiences in an incessant dopamine induced excitement that keeps viewers return for additional. Through creating niches that are based on the most extreme fantasies for instance having a relationship with an older woman or young boys, and vice versa; females who have huge boobs, Sodomy and fetish-like fantasies; long blondes wearing high heels sexual fantasies, or taboos which are not normally possible in real life This creates a lust inside you. It also triggers stimulation of your brain that is unnatural and can make you want to watch the videos over and over again.

Internet porn can be significantly more sexually stimulating as other forms of porn. It is due to the abundance of self-select access and the countless potent content available and the intense quality of the content. The modern porn user can create the sensation of erotic pleasure by clicking the novel or a new genre that will cause a greater sense of stimulation. The majority of porn addicts have developed methods to prolong or delay this experience so that they get more "kick off' from their dopamine. In a way, by putting off ejaculating or stopping videos and taking in multiple films in a row, addicts of porn prolong the dopamine cycle so that they can stay for a bit longer within their state of halo.

The result is the development of addiction and unhealthy sexual lives since, in reality it is difficult for them to be attracted or enticed by men or women since their brains and minds have been trained to get a kick out of these kinds of stimuli which are not present in reality. That's why both men and females who are married or engaged in relationships are prone to masturbating despite engaging in regular sexual activities due to the fact that their partner is not capable of stimulating them in the same manner that porn.

In her book Bunny Tales: Behind Closed Doors at the Playboy Mansion, Izabella St James, a playboy's housekeeper and among the "official girlfriends" to the host, Hugh Hefner, described sexual relations with the host. The 70-year-old Hefner enjoyed an orgy every two weeks every week with a variety of sexual friends. In the final moments, Hefner had to masturbate in front of porn, despite the an orgy. This was a person who was living his fantasies in the Eldorado in his sexual fantasies. There was novelty, variety of choice, a variety, and real porn stars who would perform whatever he wanted. You would think that all this would propel him to his sexual bliss. But, Hugh Hefner turned away towards touch and flesh to get a rush of stimulation from pictures on the screen.

The porn culture de-sensitizes its fans to less pleasurable pursuits and increases the level of sexual pleasure. When the tolerance for sexual pleasure grows, traditional porn (whatever it is) is no longer satisfying as dopamine is losing its effectiveness due to excessive stimulation. This is the reason why current porn movies are much more threatening and extreme since the threshold of porn addiction is expanding far beyond what is typical of regular sexual activity.

When you watch a "higher or more explicit, obscene video will the user be enthralled and the levels of dopamine in their blood increase. In this way, pornographic movies include explicit sexual scenes like angry sex screaming in a snarky manner on women's faces male sexuality, submissive men getting dominated by aggressive females and rape-related scenes.

One of the most likely explanations to this sexually unhealthy behavior could be it's the Coolidge Effect, which states that as time passes the desire to sexually engage will diminish when a person is a single one and rise with the introduction of a new one. The 'newness' that always increases the levels of dopamine in the brain, could manifest itself in excessive sexual behaviour and fantasies. The reason for this is that the desire for "new" things produces more adrenaline and dopamine. With porn there are endless possibilities for sexual novelty are limitless.

Video Games

In the course of a seven-day marathon gaming and a male aged 26 Chinese known as "Zhang" passed met his tragic death from an attack of the heart. The year 2009 saw a 3 month-old South Korean child, Kim Sa-rang died from malnutrition due to the fact that both parents had been spending many hours raising their virtual baby every day on the online world of. Two scenarios illustrate the detrimental effects of games on our mental health.

Because of their completely engaging nature, characterized by huge digital environments, nuanced characters, and an obsessive scoring gaming is a different source of harmful dopamine spikes throughout our brain. Designers of video games often work with psychologists to craft strategies to keep players attracted to their devices as well as consoles, joysticks, and other devices. Many of them are based to a rewards system that offers bonuses when you log into each day, awards points or boosts life levels. In the anticipation of such rewards, typically triggers the production of dopamine that invariably causes dependency.

Teenagers today are probably more prone to playing video games than previous generations since they've not just been exposed to the latest games in a much younger age and, in addition, the games provide a gateway to virtual realms, where they escape the real life.

Online multiplayer games that permit players to interact with other gamers across the world provide a unique social experience to the community online and thereby separating gamers from real life as well as human interactions. Some gamers form a strong connection to others who they play with in the virtual world. As a result the process of logging off can be much more challenging for youngsters who've formed a connection to other players in the online community.

The Washington Post reports that the study conducted in 1998 revealed how playing games increase dopamine levels in the brain by around 100 percent. This is roughly equal to the increase caused by sexual activity. The games of today have advanced rapidly from what was in play at the time of research.

Based on the findings of the study, released in Frontiers in Human Neuroscience, researchers found noticeable changes to the areas that are responsible for mental function and control of emotions following an entire week playing intense video games. The dysfunctional behavior is described to be "gaming disorder," a expression used to describe the excessive and addictive engrossing in video games that result in severe social academic, and occupational impairments for at least twelve months.

While there's a wealth of studies examining the impact of video games on our brain, some of which question their addictive and harmful impacts, one common thread that runs across these diverse findings is the capacity of games on video to stimulate the brain! A few studies have shown that playing video games help our brains to be more efficient at learning, enhance co-centration, and help develop abilities.

Chapter 4: Social Media/Smart Phones

Usually the moment we forget our phone, we're in a anxiety until the phone has located. Many people suffer from the 'phantom vibration syndrome. It's been so attached to phones that, sometimes they vibrate in our pockets, even when they're not. Mobile phones and social media platforms are transforming us into digital addicts.

The results of a study regarding the effects technological devices on the anxiety level, conducted by a group of psychologists at the California State University led by Larry Rosen found out that people check their phones at least every 15 minutes with half of the time the phone is not alerted or notifications. In an article from 2017 published by The New York Times titled 'How evil is technology? writer David Brooks opined that technology firms understand the causes of dopamine spikes in our brains and infuse their products with "attention-grabbing techniques which entice us and draw us in to a state of compulsion.

Smartphones give us a plethora of amount of social stimulation that are both negative and positive. Every alert, be it as a text message, like, or comment has the capacity to trigger. It is a compulsion to constantly look up our comments and likes in the form of comments on Instagram or Facebook or emails, and then respond to them or even looking forward to a phone call will likely be stimulated by the production of dopamine.

Neuroscientists who study the effect of social media on our brain have discovered that even positive social interactions, such as the person who likes your blog post is likely to trigger the exact sort of chemical response that can be triggered by gambling or recreational drug. Utilizing social media, or simply surfing on the internet mimics exact same type of stimulant that you get by smoking cigarettes, alcohol, as well as other drugs. The scientific evidence suggests that we carry tiny doses of dopamine within our pockets.

In a report published in 2018 written by Harvard University researcher, Trevor Haynes When you receive notifications from social media sites the brain releases dopamine, which can make you feel happy. That's why social media is rapidly becoming the center of narcissism. It is common for people to do something that goes viral in order to gain an increase in followers, likes or likes. They feel that they need others to affirm them and their actions. They're like addicts searching for the next shot of dopamine. In addition, the article states that around 73% of the population feel anxious while looking at their phone.

The reward centers of our brains get the most engaged when we're chatting about our own lives. Social media provides the ideal opportunity to display our self-esteem and showcase our life. If someone receives a favorable review from a post or comment published, it triggers neurons to produce dopamine for reward. This further reinforces the process of sharing and seeking feedback. This is the reason why social media can be the source of Narcissism.

How can social media businesses make the most of dopamine-driven behaviors? Like betting shops and casinos, social media companies employ rewards that are created to engage users in the most immersive way feasible. In a conversation in The Guardian, Sean Parker who was the founder of Facebook said that Facebook was created not with the intention of uniting users, but rather to divert the users. "The initial thought was "How do we consume the most time and attention as is possible?

Facebook, Twitter, Snapchat as well as Instagram as well as the rest of them rely their dopamine-driven beginnings that are used by casinos porn websites videos, casinos, as well as hard drugs, to keep users to their social media platforms for as long as they can. The question is if they're intended to assist people in living their lives? Are they designed for the purpose of luring customers to use the item? A thorough look at the science behind them could make your mind pause the next time you feel that pockets vibrate.

As an example, Facebook uses a continuous scroll in their feeds because it's a tried and tested method to keep you entertained as you continue scrolling in order to browse for a longer period of time. Instagram is, on the contrary however, utilizes its notifications algorithm to keep users glued. The method is to withhold "likes" on your photos or counting visits to your profile that are then delivered with massive volumes. In other words the moment you post an Instagram post, you might find yourself disappointed to receive fewer reactions than what you expected but then get the responses in greater numbers afterward. However, it is likely that the disappointment earlier caused you to make more posts in the future on Instagram. Snapchat's streak which displays the amount of days that the user can send a message to someone is also based in the same way. To catch-up, Snapchat users who aren't willing to let their streak' will continue sending messages in a back and forth.

The dopamine systems in your brain are activated in response to those first negative results or delaying strategies for you to respond quickly to the incoming flood of social appraising. A few programmers have termed the process in the context of "brain hacking." With social media, the internet as well as messaging applications immediate satisfaction of the desire for validation is just a mouse click away. Chatting is only a click or a call away. The it takes just a couple of seconds. You only need a single click for all the info you'd like. This makes it easy for smartphone users to be sucked hooked into a dopamine-induced cycle which makes you search and be rewarded for it as well as invariably make you want to seek out even more. In this way, it's hard to keep a check on notifications from your smartphone.

Alcohol

Alcohol consumption doesn't just reduce the self-esteem of our clients, but it also directly alters the brain's structure. As per the World Health Organization, dependence of alcohol affects around 140 million people worldwide and is one of the major causes for the worldwide burden of illness. It's the fifth most significant danger factor in premature deaths and disabilities among alcoholics.

In the event of drinking alcohol, our reward circuits in the brain are filled with dopamine and create an incredibly powerful impact. The more alcohol we consume and the more powerful the effect as our dopamine receptors get affected. In the end, nothing can get your mind ready for another drink like the taste of a beer.

In the beginning, alcohol consumption increases the dopamine levels in your brain. When drinking alcohol is consumed continuously that the brain adapts to the increased levels of dopamine. After it, begins to release lesser amount of dopamine. It is accomplished by decreasing the amount of dopamine receptors within the body as well as expanding the dopamine transporters that help to eliminate the excessive amount of dopamine stored in brain cells.

When the dopamine level in our brains decreases, so do our moods. As a result, we drink more alcohol to restore our "spark and vigor back. Proficient drinkers understand the most effective way to boost your spirits if you are suffering from a hangover is by drinking the time to drink a glass of wine

The latest research in science sheds more light on the relation between dopamine and addiction to alcohol. The research has shown that individuals with the family heritage of alcohol dependence are at a greater risk to become addicted because they were born with an enlargement of Dopamine receptors D2. They are dopamine-friendly, or "no-go" receptors (the other one being D1 (also known as "go" receptors), which block the messages.

Balance between two receptors (D1 and D2) aids in keeping the desire to take another drink within control. When there's an ongoing intake of alcohol (or other stimulants like alcohol or other stimulants like drugs), D2 receptors tend to become deactivated. It reduces the inhibition of drinking alcohol, which causes us to drink more as there's no inhibition to self-control.

In order to test the impact of weak D2 receptors on behaviour, researchers of the Alcohol Research Center of Indiana University have trained the mice to show the resemblance of alcoholics, by placing them through an experiment of alcohol-related binge drinking sessions and recovering. Unsurprisingly, the identical D2 receptors located in the brain displayed indications of less activity, which suggests that the mice experienced more compelled to consume alcohol. The researchers then altered the receptors in order to see what the mice's reactions were. Intensifying the activities of D2 receptors caused mice to drink less, whereas increasing the D1 receptors made them consume more. Through small changes in their nervous system researchers were able to regulate mouse's addiction behaviors, giving explanations of similar behavior in human beings.

This research explains how difficult it can be for people who are alcoholics to leave. They are not only attracted by feelings of pleasure and pleasure, but their inhibitions have gone away. Through stimulating the release of dopamine inside your brain, alcohol can create a trick that allows you to believe you're feeling good. In the end, you drink more to gain greater dopamine levels, however in the process changing certain brain chemicals that could hinder the ability of you to indulge in this behaviour.

Chapter 5: Drugs

Drugs that are hard to get can trigger 10 times or more the quantity of dopamine that is released in the case of eating food or having sexual arousal. The continuous use of substances causes the brain to create the hormone transfusing, releasing, and then sponge in less dopamine and leading to a change in the chemical balance within the brain. The mind-altering drugs flood the brain with massive quantities of dopamine that is usually not absorbed in a normal manner. The result is a huge amount of dopamine found in the brain all in a single moment.

Dopamine's surge triggers an euphoria-like feeling and can make us get "high." This supposedly enjoyable feeling can make users want to replicate the experience by resuming their drug usage. Similar to the other substances of abuse described earlier, after the effects of a drug diminish the levels of dopamine decrease which triggers distressing withdrawal symptoms, as well as intense cravings. Users are then in a need to continue using drugs in order to prevent the signs and urges as dependency develops.

But, despite the intense feeling of satisfaction and anticipation of benefits derived from the use of drugs play a significant role in reviving the cycle of abuse and dependence and addiction, they are only a small part of the neurophysiological system that triggers addiction. As opposed to normal reward stimulations like food and sexual stimulation, the excessive stimulation of dopamine, which mind-altering substances create doesn't stop naturally after the reward has been obtained. The desire for rewards that come with the drug continue to happen regardless of the drug used that invariably leads into a habitual, repeated usage. Like alcohol, it reduces the amount of dopamine receptors within the brain, as it attempts to adapt to the increased levels of dopamine.

A more serious and damaging consequence of a long-term use of drugs can be seen in the drastic changes to the human behaviour it's likely to cause, usually time with detrimental consequences to individual health, life in general as well as society at large. Regular cocaine users battle to manage their emotions taking decisions when they should, and performing basic motor functions even after having abstained from using the drug. The use of marijuana in teenagers and early adulthood depletes the of brain grey matter and can cause long-term mental and behavioral problems. The habitual consumption of Methamphetamine may damage as much as half the dopamine producing cells that make up the brain.

This kind of harm from drugs can cause a profound modification to the brain's functioning structures, resulting in problems with memory and learning difficulties, psychosis anger, depression as well as Parkinson's disease. The meth-related effects that are sometimes reversed, last for a long time when abstinence is not achieved.

In the event of addiction, it can be difficult to experience pleasure in regular actions. Through an experiment on laboratory rats, researchers discovered that the feeling of joy that drugs provide was so intense that the rats were able to give up food and die to get high. In the absence of any interaction with the drugs, users experience an anxiety-related depression, insomnia, and stress and restlessness. and cognitive impairment. A lot of the harm resulted from drug use is reversed by prolonged absence from drugs; however, certain of the adverse symptoms may take a while to heal completely.

Gambling

If gamblers place their money to the test, they experience an "thrill." Those who gamble regularly recognize that the time the wheels spin is the time when you feel an overwhelming excitement. When you gamble, your reward system in the brain to release greater than what naturally satisfying experiences could produce.

As the brain gets used to massive doses of dopamine levels, gamblers are able to establish the threshold for tolerance that increases as they continue to indulge. The reason for this is that the dopamine release does not produce the similar "thrill" as it did at first, causing the brain produce an increase in dopamine. The brain's reward system, and ultimately lowers the degree of "pleasure" the individual experiences. In turn, the brain is conditioned, and it longs for more dopamine that triggers the reward system.

Most of the time, gamblers prefer to gamble in order to win. This is why, even after massive wins, when you'd anticipate them to shut shop and eat their gains and leave the ship gambling addicts continue to return to play the games, machines and races. The financial rewards are seen as a chance to increase the time of play, as opposed to achieving the principal goal. It is true that losing money could motivate gamblers more than winnings is also hard to comprehend.

Research has shown that gamblers with compulsive tendencies and drug addicts share a similar tendency to impulse and craving for rewards. Like substance addicts need more powerful hits to be high, gamblers who are compulsive are more prone to risky ventures. Uncertain rewards is the main reason why they run the mill.

American psychology B.F. Skinner, who is well-known for his pioneering research into the psychology of motivation and behavior, believes that the best way to reinforce the behavior you have learned is by rewarding it with an unplanned schedule. Feeling euphoric after playing the game and taking risk is the reward for gamblers. The feeling of elation, not the money is what drives people to gamble.

The dope is removed from dopamine

When you reach the goal and make money, reach the goal, seal the deal or ascend to an enviable position You experience a surge of dopamine. This will make you want to do more. It's true that you can succeed, and then it wears off creating a desire for greater success, money, or even more power.

Dopamine, the primary fuel source that fuels ambitious individuals that encourages covetousness and greed as well as a sense of importance. Dopamine can even lead to outbreaks of war and even pestilence. It would be a bit inappropriate to claim that Hitler was fueled by dopamine? It would be a derogatory statement to suggest that all of dictators are brimming with dopamine? The ones who seek influence, popularity or power aren't any different than drug addicts or those who drink. The aspiring athlete or committed scientist is not any different than a child holding his gaming device or gambling. These are all powered by dopamine differently.

Dopamine enhances the future use of resources. It can put one in an dreamlike mental state. It causes us to be nervous, elated as well as excited and optimistic. This chemical is known as a pleasure one. the world a more peaceful environment.

Dopamine acts as a catalyst to altruism and encourages us to make improvements in ourselves and our environment. Dopamine inspired a young child who saw injustice into becoming an attorney for civil rights so that he could assist those who were in need. Dopamine motivates individuals to become firefighters, teachers, policemen as well as other such. Dopamine allows us to dream goals and pursue these desires.

In order to determine the significance of dopamine in body's research psychologists at University of Michigan. University of Michigan destroyed dopamine neurons in rats. Researchers discovered that even though rats were able to walk through the food chain, chew, and swallow their food, they lost the desire and anticipation for food. Many were starving to death, even in the presence of food right before their eyes.

Dopamine drives athletes to be the best in what they do. Swedish legend Zlatan Ibrahimovic, was driven to be the top player due to his lack of and rocky background. Tupac was motivated to fame by the sufferings and injustices that his African-American community faced and incorporated them into his music; that's the reason he was the greatest ever rapper. Muhammad Ali was motivated because his instructor told him the amount he could make was insignificant. In the event that he won an Olympic silver medal for boxing Ali gave it to the teacher whom he told he'd be nothing. I am convinced that Elon Musk's motivation is dopamine in connection with his goal of creating reusable rockets which could take us on a trip to space.

Everything that makes you feel fantasies or provides you with an escape to reality dopamine-rich. However, many of us turn into vices in order to boost dopamine levels. This is evident from these cases causes addiction that has wider impact on our overall health.

Dopamine in its own way isn't a bad thing since it allows us to reach the goals we set for ourselves. It helps us to have the drive and motivation to do better and get better over ourselves. There are many natural methods to stimulate the release of dopamine. Exercises as well as healthy sexual routines that are controlled, ambition-controlled, and even love are a few methods that are healthy to increase our levels of dopamine. But the key is keeping the amount in check so that it doesn't lead us to addiction.

But, dopamine may also cause harm. Dopamine's excessive release can cause psychological instability which can cause the loss of any passion, motivation or goal-directed behaviour. Dopamine levels are elevated when you stimulate it. the amount of joy, satisfaction or happiness rises and, in the majority of cases can't be sustained by reality. It raises the level of your personal happiness. This means that you'll are always in need of more the hits that make you feel happy, joyful, so that you can enjoy the reward. It's much more difficult to be content, happy as well as alive and enthusiastic. When people overload themselves, their neurotransmitters go in a state of imbalance that makes them are numb. People feel depressed, which can lead to depression, anxiety or addiction as well as a loss of enthusiasm. They are all fueled by dopamine.

This is where the fear comes in. In the event that you are trying to end the excessive stimulation of your life, such as the consumption of alcohol, pornography or binge-watching films, sugar or playing video games, you will experience withdrawal symptoms. These are when things become worse before they get improved. The severity of depression increases when you experience intense anxiety and anxiety, stress, or worry. This means that the same signs that fuel your desire for dopamine surge increase in intensity in the beginning as you decrease the amount of dopamine you get. That's why the majority of individuals return to their natural forms of pleasure which they feel a connection to as they lack the mental strength to endure the awe of withdrawal.

The thing we have observed in people who engage heavily in dopamine-driven behaviours (natural and non-natural) is that they can be disguised as an underlying psychological issue. Dopamine-driven hits can be employed to hide the emotions of others or to cover up issues aren't resolved. We seek to get our attention with the dopamine rush in order to keep us from being distracted. This is an instinctive human nature. If we face difficulties or problems We tend to take the easiest route to get out of it and often is not the ideal choice. When we experience the symptoms mentioned above, we switch off with binge watching videos and surfing the internet, or using drugs or playing the lottery. These vices are embraced due to the way our bodies feel. We are trying to relieve ourselves from feelings of boredom emptyness, stress, or boredom. But, if you constantly cover up your feelings or feeling of stress to escape to avoid problems, you create more obstacles within our lives. It's like quicksand. If you are trying to break free and out, the deeper you get into.

With this in mind it is possible to find ways in to detoxify dopamine's surge within the brain, and then stop the addiction. Other neurotransmitters could be developed to help balance the excessive stimulation of dopamine. Additionally, there are traits are attainable to imbibe and help to counteract the negative effects of the dopamine surge. What is essential is perseverance, mental toughness, and the desire to persevere until the very end. There's no shortcut to fame.

Here & Now

A way to eliminate dopamine is by development of 'Here and Now neurotransmitters. Endorphins and serotonin as well as oxytocin and Gamma-aminobutyric acids GABA are neurotransmitters which allow users to be in the now. The brain's chemicals are responsible for processing things that impact us within the present, or our social space. If the brain is processing things that are outside of our personal space, it utilizes dopamine.

Interaction with other things in an personal space happens in the near future since these items aren't happening now. For instance, you imagine what you would accomplish if we won one million dollars; or we win the job we have been battling to get. These desires do not have a tangible form. They are concepts abstract that are a part of our mind. They're fictitious and they aren't real. Dopamine can be described as the chemical that gives us the things we want. The brain's equilibrium as well as our mental wellbeing depends on how well we manage both of these spaces, without overturning the balance scale.

The neurotransmitters in the present enable you to experience tranquility, happiness and appreciate the time. Neurotransmitters like these are those we can count on to provide lasting happiness and happiness throughout our lives. Through here and now chemicals, we are able to feel happiness, sadness, and joy. The five senses also get activated by these and other chemical substances. The senses are triggered by emotions of warmth, empathy and the pure joy sharing time with those who you cherish in this moment. They are chemical compounds that interact in our interactions with other people.

Today, neurotransmitters are what allow us to have more stability in our relationships and give us an overall view of life as well as help us focus on the details and also help to avoid the chaos which is the norm in this society. It is the reason why certain couples can't stand each other for two years, some couples still share the same spark fifty years later when they first began dating. That's why, even if you haven't achieved your ideal status or achieved the success he desires, he's happy and takes pleasure in enjoying the moment. The neurotransmitters are a source of peace for the mind even in conflict. Therefore, they must be cultivated and nurtured for us to live in this moment in time and enjoy lasting peace in our lives.

In reality, most of the good aspects that happen in our lives are located within that Here and Now. In the case of sex, for instance, we be tempted to engage in sex for high on dopamine and stimulate our body. But, things as simple as making a song, writing poems, taking an outing with loved family members, or engaging engaged in healthy discussions can work as healthy alternatives to lust-driven sexual activities.

Chapter 6: Slow, Gradual And Calculated Withdrawal

Another approach to lessen the brain's desire to reward itself is by a gradual, slow and controlled withdrawal of the behavioral habits that cause us to crave dopamine. In the case of frequently engage in sexual activity, you can cut it down by only masturbating within two days. Then, gradually increase the amount. If you're a smoker every day, you could make an effort to lessen smoking it twice every day or even once. If you're a sex fan and aren't satisfied with having a sexy time You can search for additional characteristics that will increase the attractiveness of your partner to you different from sexual intimacy. Look for those who are able to keep your attention with stimulating conversation.

The most important thing is to take a steady method of recovering your mental and physical stability. Be aware that if you attempt to take the effects of dopamine which you've depended on for a long time without thinking about it, you will be re-inducing the same effect into a far more aggressive manner.

There is the option of choosing certain days of the week where you don't engage in these activities. Choose a day on the weekend that allows your mind to relax. Simply be in the moment without thinking about anything or let anything worry you. You can choose to go for a 30-day duration, or a week or even 90 days. This is contingent the intensity of by your dopamine level and how long you're willing for detoxification. In some cases, it could take some time for the brain to reset or rewire your baseline level to return to normal. That's typical with the use of hard drugs.

Meditate

One of the most important things to bring us to the present current moment is the practice of meditation. Meditation is a vital necessity in the present since we're constantly bombarded with a myriad of issues that are competing for our focus. Meditation is a dual approach. While it is a method to reduce healthy dopamine levels within our brains caused by stress, depression or even anger It can also be employed to increase dopamine levels naturally by focusing on happiness, optimism and breath deep. It stimulates the reward system even without any stimulant to the mind.

The trick is to give your mind empty that is free of thoughts. Focus on what is happening in the moment and not think about any other thought. It puts you at the top of a mountain to face the problems that life throws at us. The calmness of our minds allows us to confront the turbulence of life, and not look for escape routes.

The majority of people are struggling when they meditate because their brains become over-stimulated and this causes distracting thoughts. Meditation can help you get your brain back in order and decreases the level of your base. It helps you build your strength to fight off temptations that result through the cravings for dopamine. If you are unable to meditate for 10 minutes this means that your brain is blocked by over-analyzing and excessive stimulation.

Self-Reflect

One of the most effective methods to live at the present moment is to imagine your thoughts look like a mirror. Mirrors refuse to accept nothing, yet is unable to grasp anything. It takes whatever you can throw at it however, it doesn't own it. Therefore, try to be able to grab absolutely nothing. Whatever life may throw at you simply be present at the present moment and avoid being awed by the moment. Bruce Lee referred to this state of mindlessness as Wu-Shin. where the mind is free to move with no inhibitions, stress or stress.

Therefore, instead of having a fervent desire to achieve success, gain money or find love, why not be a mere existence? Stay in the moment. Instead of trying to get rid of the emotional pain or blame the past, parents or even your own acquaintances for the problems you've faced Why don't you view your experience as a process of learning to improve your character?

Life is a circular thing and is not a straight line It is full of both ups and downs. But when you look at it from a different angle, one see the positivity of each experience, no matter how positive or negative. Even the good as well as bad mental constructs and are based on the way we perceive our circumstances. Be flexible and don't suffocate your feelings as dams. Infuse Bruce Lee's famous quote. Like water. When water is put into a container, it changes shape to match the cup. If it is then put into a container, it is shaped like the Jar. However, it does not change its fundamental value being water. The circumstances shouldn't be the sole determinant of who you are since If they do, you'll need to get out using gaming, drugs, or by creating a persona through social media.

Question Your Habits

It is also possible to make new choices that stimulate your brain in a healthy way. dopamine. They serve as a replacement for the older habits, which have affected your brain's dopamine receptors with harmful ways. If you take away from the previous habit, without substituting it with a new one, you're likely to fall back into habit in an violent approach. As you attempt to get rid of the habit of masturbation, try immersing yourself in a brand new habit or mastering something new whenever you have the desire. It's as easy as staying far from the phone or going on a walk or acquiring the language of your choice could be the answer. What's important is that you must find something new to do and keep your mind off engaging in unhealthy habits.

Seek out Companionship

You should have a partner or professional who will guide you through the steps. Self-actualization and self-discovery is often a dangerous and lonely. In this regard, you may require someone to talk to or a friend who will keep you accountable and track your daily progress. Similar to your parole agent who makes sure that you do not get over the edge. It is possible to find someone who are able to trust when it comes to your feelings as well as your fears and anxieties and then let him or her guide you along the way.

Additionally, discussing or sharing stories can help. Sharing experiences can make a difference. solved. It is possible that we carry the burden within our bodies unaware there are others who suffer similar issues or greater. Conversation can help reduce stress and anxiety and helps us focus on the ways we can seek aid. There's an Igbo Proverb which states that anyone who asks questions doesn't get lost.

Increase your circle of friends

Have more fun with your friends. Maintain a balanced social life. Social interaction with others builds connections as well as intimacy. It helps us feel present. Many of the items that trigger the rush of dopamine cause us to be withdrawn because they keep are a distraction from the people that we cherish. In turn when we engage in these activities it is the more we get attracted to them since we are prone to connect to only those who are able to share the same values as us.

It is important to have a social and enjoyable life. We should be able to mix with those outside of our friends who are prone to the same addictions as we do. It helps us break the dependency of negatives, and allows us to discover different ways to live and living with a more balanced mind. To follow up to this, we should beware of environments and situations that encourage unhealthful pleasure seeking habits. Avoiding scenarios that may cause us to be a victim, we can increase the likelihood of avoiding the same things.

Enjoy Nature

Additionally, take time to enjoy nature. In love with the natural world. Go for walks. Relax and enjoy the refreshing air as well as the stability of trees, and the calmness of the animals. Take a bath in the beauty of your environment. Pay attention to what you eat.

If you're looking to be successful It is recommended to start releasing the dopamine in your brain. But, once you've reached your goals and that unanticipated reward is realized, it is important to redirect your energy elsewhere to avoid it being destroyed as if you were to open a dam, which lets water out into the quantum.

Chapter 7: Dopamine And Its Major Roles

Dopamine is an organic molecule which is part of the chemical same family the catecholamines as well as the phenethylamines. It is involved in regulating your central nervous system. Dopamine is an important neurotransmitter. Dopamine is an instance of a neurotransmitter. It is a chemical which transmits signals across the nervous system.

Dopaminergic signaling is associated with both behaviour which is motivated by reward and motor control. In addition, disturbances in the dopamine systems have been associated with several diseases. Dopaminergic signaling is also associated with motor control. There is also evidence that dopaminergic signals are involved in regulating motion. A form of Parkinson's disease called degenerative Parkinson's disease is defined by the demise of the neurons accountable for the release of dopamine. Dopamine eventually causes motor impairment. The pathology can be directly linked to the demise of the neurons responsible for producing dopamine.

Dopamine. Are you in a position to inform me on the subject? For more precise information what region in the brain that is responsible for performing the functions?

Dopamine is a type of neurotransmitter which brains are able to produce independently. Its most basic function it performs its function of being an electronic messenger between neurons. A different method of saying the fact that it is able to perform that role.

Dopamine can be described as a neurotransmitter which gets released into bloodstream in the event that the individual's brain anticipates receiving an reward. In anticipation, the brain is triggered to create an increase in dopamine.

If you've trained your brain to connect an activity to happy memories, then the mere desire to engage in that activity could be enough to result in an increase in amount of dopamine that you have within the brain. This could be due to a particular sort of cuisine, sex shopping, or everything else you enjoy engaging in during your leisure moments. Your ideals could be something you love. It is possible that it's something completely different.

Consider, for example for instance, that the most frequently used "comfort food" consists of homemade, baked two chocolate chips. If you can smell something in the kitchen or look at something recently cooked out of the oven the brain might create more dopamine than it normally does. It can happen after you detect the smell of cooking food or observe the food. The desire to eat food will become greater due to the dopamine surge generated after you consume these foods, as well as in the future, you'll likely to pay more your energy on satisfying it.

Positive cycles include activities like encouraging, rewarding, or encouraging the positive behavior of another individual.

Imagine looking for the cookies you wanted, but when you were in the phone, you colleagues ate all of them prior to you having the chance to grab some for yourself as they were distracted by calling. The likelihood is that your frustration causes a decline in the amount of dopamine you're releasing and cause your mood more miserable. This could be an endless cycle. Furthermore it is possible that this will boost the desire for chocolate chip double cookies. Are you still in the market for these cookies, despite being aware that you crave these cookies higher than previously?

Dopamine can be found in many various activities in the human body. It is also involved in its function in the creation of what's typically called"a "good feeling." A few examples can be found below:

* Blood flow

* Digestion

* Ability to form views on matters that concern high-ranking officials in the company

* The health of the kidneys in the patient's body and cardiovascular system

Engaging in deep thought or focusing one's focus

* The emotional and mental condition of the person who is in the question

* Motor control

The management of an unpleasant physical sensation

Control of the production of insulin and its secretion as well as the general function of the pancreas.

* A mindset that is driven by satisfaction and satisfaction in all one's endeavours

* Sleep

* The stress response

It is crucial to bear the fact that dopamine as it is, on its own does not perform its regular tasks. It performs this function by engaging in chemical exchanges that involve a diverse array of neurotransmitters and hormones such adrenaline and serotonin, which are required to produce the result which is required.

Your environment being in impacts not only on your mental and physical well-being, but also various other aspects of your daily life, and the manner in which you lead it.

Dopamine is also known as 3, 4-dihydroxytyramine is the subject of an extensive amount of studies since it was first recognized. It's due to the nature of dopamine being the very first neurotransmitter that was found. It's composed of a benzene circle that includes two side groups of hydroxyl that are linked and linked with a hydroxyl cluster. Additionally, it's linked by a hydroxyl group. Following that the ethyl group utilized to join these side groups of hydroxyl to the amine groups. In the end, the product is an amine. Dopamine is made by Tyrosine, an amino acid that is produced in dopaminergic neurons located in the brain. The process begins by the addition of a hydroxyl molecule, that transforms to L-DOPA (or Levo-DOPA) by removing an acid carboxylic group of an ethyl side chain, which is linked to the amine molecule that result in dopamine. The process is repeated several times until adequate amount of dopamine is created. Dopaminergic neurons can be located in 3 different areas of the brain, including the substantia-nigra region, the ventral tegmental region and the arcuate nucleus in the hypothalamus. The specific neurons that are found in these regions are those within the brain which have the responsibility for the creation of this chemical that signals the body. It is generally accepted that each of these areas are part of the brain's midbrain. Dopamine is known as a neurotransmitter meaning that it's the substance secreted by neurons to aid in the transmission of the electrical signals from one nerve to the one next to transmit information from and to in the central nervous system. Dopamine is a chemical which helps neurons connect with one another. Dopamine is an neurotransmitter which helps to facilitate communications between neurons. As such, it is essential to the overall health of brain cells. Dopamine is one of the neurotransmitters and is transported into synaptic vasoconsicle by the vesicular monamine transporter 2 (VMAT2). Then, it is stored in the vesicles till action potentials cause the release of dopamine in the synaptic cleft, and trigger the binding of dopamine receptors to the neurons that are postsynaptic. The dopamine-producing process is first initiated, and then the process described following it.

Dopamine is one of the neurotransmitters and is involved in a range of crucial tasks in the human brain.

Dopamine is a key component in motor control, executive functions as well as motivation, arousal reinforcement and reward through the through signaling cascades which can be triggered through the binding of dopaminergic receptors to projections within the substantia nigra and ventral tegmental region as well as the arcuate nucleus in the hypothalamus of our brains. The projections can be found within the substantia nigra as well as the ventral tegmental space as well as

Dopaminergic neurons are located in the area that is the source of input for the substantia nerve, which can also be referred to the pars compacta. The nigrostriatal pathway is located within the area of the substantia nigra and connects these neuronal into the dorsal part of the striatum. The nigro-striatal pathway is of crucial importance for controlling motor functions as well as for the development of motor skills that are not previously known. The abnormal regulation of motor function is one key characteristics that define Parkinson's disease. The disorder can come due to the decline of dopaminergic nerves in the nigrostriatal path that is among those pathways implicated in the disease.

The ventral tegmental area and the nucleus accumbens region of the amygdala hippocampus, cingulate gyrus and the pyriform system of the olfactory bulbs are all associated with the mesolimbic pathway (VTA). The mesolimbic pathway began within the cortex of prefrontal, and extends to the ventral-thalamic region (VTA). The development of feelings and the processing of these emotions are affected by dopaminergic projections within the amygdala as well as the Cingulate Gyrus. It is known there is a presence of dopaminergic neuron in the hippocampus can be linked to processes related to learning, the formation of memory in working memory as well as the creation of memory in the long-term storage. The pyriform component of the olfactory bulb allows people to smell. This leads us to our last aspect. The olfactory bulbs is the home to this complex network of structure. Dopamine releases from mesolimbic pathways when situations seem to be enjoyable. This causes arousal and influences behaviour (motivations) and causes people to search for activities that are enjoyable or work. Dopaminergic receptors are present in both the nucleus of accumbens and in the prefrontal cortex, may be influenced by it. Reinforcing the process addiction, and stronger forms of addiction is caused by increased activity projections towards the nucleus of Acumbens. It has a significant role to play.

The formation of the tuberoinfundibular path results from the activities of dopamine neuron, which reside in the arcuate nucleus within the hypothalamus. The pathway leads into the pituitary gland in which it fulfills its purpose of blocking the production of hormone called prolactin. The neurons located within the arcuate nucleus are the ones responsible for the production of dopamine. This hormone is released into the blood vessels found within the hypothalamus and hypophysis. These blood vessels provide the pituitary glands with dopamine which limits the prolactin production. The process is referred to as feedback loop.

Chapter 8: Quantitative Methods For Assessing The Dopamine Levels In Selected Samples

Dopamine levels and the misregulation of certain processes linked to regions of the brain have been of great interest for researchers working within the field of neuroscience as one of the aims in this field of study is to discover the connection between these two. The highly sensitive test has an ability to detect a range of levels that allow it to determine concentrations between 1.56 to 1.0 ng/ml and all the way up to 100 mg/ml. It's able to recognize these concentrations due to its ability to find quantities that are very low or extremely high. Additionally, the product has been designed to have high sensitivity and high reproducibility from lot to lot and a quick time-to-result. it offers a simple procedure that produces precise, accurate results to our customers within less than 2 hours, spread over 24 hours or more.

Dopamine is one of the neurotransmitters and is responsible for a range of impacts on our bodies.

You may have heard that someone said that dopamine, a neurotransmitter, is what causes that "feel good" emotion. There are many connections to be made between these two.

Dopamine, the neurotransmitter in our brains, is associated with feelings of satisfaction and satisfaction. Naturally, there's more to this than can be understood by looking at that basic description. Actually there's a whole quantity more to this intricate chemical process than was previously mentioned.

Dopamine plays a role in the workings in the nerve system, in conjunction with the function of the other body systems. This is an aspect which affects more than just the ability of our body to move but also the state of our thoughts and the choices we make. Furthermore the fact that it is associated with various mental and motor problems.

Dopamine plays a number of functions In this piece we will look at some functions, and the signs that may occur in the event that your body doesn't possess sufficient dopamine.

How do you feel?

We know that having a good dose of dopamine leads to an attitude which is described as highly positive. This is a great way to boost efficiency, and also for plans and education.

Dopamine can be described as a neurotransmitter and can be found in a broad spectrum of feelings, including the ability to focus, alertness as well as motivation and happiness. Dopamine can also play a role as a reward mechanism in the brain.

Dopamine's infusion has the capability of creating brief emotions of happiness. However, these feelings can only be temporary.

Are you able to tell if there is a deficiency in dopamine?

It's likely that the levels of dopamine in your body are low. This could be one reason why you're not in a good present. You could experience some of the symptoms listed below: less concentration, alertness or concentrating, less enthusiasm and motivation as well as poor coordination and problems moving.

There's a good chance that if you're sleeping too little Dopamine levels in your body are likely to drop.

It's possible that the absence of dopamine could be what's making you feel tired, however it's also possible your sleeping pattern is the reason your dopamine levels fall. Both possibilities could be possible.

If you're not getting enough rest, you may see a marked decrease in the quantity of dopamine receptors awake in the morning.

Dopamine deficiency can expose a person to risk to develop a range of diseases.

Researchers have found a link with low levels of dopamine and various disorders, which include:

* Parkinson's disease. It is diagnosed by tremors and the slowing of movements, and occasionally psychosis as a sign. * Alzheimer's disease that is characterized by loss of memory.

*Depression, defined as melancholy and sleeplessness and experiencing changes in the brain as well as mania. It is caused by extreme and inexplicably high enthusiasm;

Dopamine transporter deficiency syndrome, often known as DTDS: This condition, which causes anomalies in movement that are similar to those observed in Parkinson's disease, is also known as infantile parkinsonism-dystonia. The majority of cases affect children.

What negative effects could excess dopamine can have on your body?

If your dopamine levels have risen dramatically and you are experiencing the sensation that you're in the top of your game for a short time. Furthermore you could also experience the ability to put you in an extreme state of overload.

It is possible to contribute to depression when utilized to a large extent, but only if:

* Hallucinations

* Delusions

Researchers have discovered a link to high levels of dopamine neurotransmitter and a number of illnesses and conditions that include obesity, addiction and schizophrenia.

What effect can medications have on the level of dopamine the body produces?

There's a chance that certain medications may interfere with dopamine in the way that leads to dependence in people taking the drugs.

The substances that are addictive including alcohol, nicotine or certain pharmaceuticals, are able to stimulate the dopamine system. This cycle may also be invigorated by physical exercises.

They are able to create a burst of dopamine, which is much faster and more strong than the rush is felt when you eat these choc chip doubles. The desire for more, due to its strength that you'd like it to occur as quickly as it is possible.

The brain can self-adjust the amount of dopamine produced as it gets to an amount at which it becomes a habit that becomes automated. To ensure that you experience the same amount of pleasure that was previously enjoyed, a higher amount of dopamine will be required in the near future.

Dopamine receptors are overactivated that cause reduction in the interest for other aspects of our lives, has been proven to cause negative effects on the receptors. This could result in you engaging more frequently. The ability to avoid the consumption of these substances is deteriorating rapidly.

In the event that your participation in the behaviour involved changes to being driven by desire, to being driven in a more impulsive need to feel satisfied, the addiction is taking the control. If you attempt to quit smoking cigarettes and vice versa, you are at chance of suffering from withdrawal, that could cause physical as well as mental signs.

Although you may not have utilized the chemicals in quite a while simply having the same surroundings with them could rekindle your desire to utilize the substances, putting at risk the possibility of sliding back to old habits.

The dopamine receptor plays part in the creation of addictions however, there are many additional factors that can be a factor. Alongside these aspects that are mentioned above, there are plenty of other factors involved including genetics, as well as external factors.

How do hormones impact the level of dopamine produced in the body?

Dopamine is capable of connecting to a range of neurotransmitters and hormones thanks to its distinctive communications capabilities. One example is glutamate, a neurotransmitter that plays a role in the reward and pleasure circuit of the brain.

The results of the research show that testosterone, estrogen and glucocorticoids interact in a way and play an effect on the level of dopamine. In the teens through the adulthood stage, it could affect the development of the brain, as well as the functioning of cognitive processes.

There are a myriad of elements of the environment which could affect neurotransmitters. The results presented by scientists suggest that the hormones produced by sexual activity have been found to be "deeply associated" with the neurotransmitters below: dopamine serotonin glutamate

The fact that they are complex is an understatement. There is only a sliver of knowledge about them. It is imperative to conduct more research in order to be able to grasp a full understanding of how dopamine is interacted with various other hormones and neurotransmitters within the body.

You must know the most important information be aware of regarding dopamine withdrawal

Dopamine detoxing requires people to work hard to remove themselves from the intense stimulation which is an everyday aspect of their lives including sweets, social media and shopping. These are discarded in favour of routines and life decisions that require smaller, more spontaneous decisions for the person. The amount of time an individual decides to refrain from eating is completely dependent on them. It could be a matter that lasts a few hours or something like several days.

It is of paramount importance to remember that dopamine detoxification is not a therapy which has been studied in a scientific setting. This is a crucial aspect to consider. There is no evidence to suggest that there are potential benefits can be found in anecdotes, and a majority of advantages stem from not taking part in activities that carry the possibility of becoming addictive. (Citation required) On the contrary there isn't a single instance of these activities is related to being dopamine-free within the strictest definition of the word.

This isn't backed by any scientifically credible study that overly simplifies the functioning of the brain. Furthermore, the concept of completing an "dopamine detox" in its entirety isn't supported by a significant research study. (Case in Point: (Case in Point:) [Case in Point:] [Case of the moment [Case] The current pattern that is referred to as "dopamine detox" gives the perception that the issue can be solved much more easily as opposed to it being; but this isn't an actual fact.

Chapter 9: Does A Dopamine Detox Work?

To fully detoxify the dopamine system, an person must refrain from all things that produce dopamine for some time. The duration could range from an hour up to a few days, based on the extent of the problem. The length of time required for treatment of an individual could differ, based on the severity of their condition.

For a successful detox of dopamine, it's essential that the person stay away from any type of stimulation, including ones that have a connection to the pleasure-inducing triggers. This is essential when you are in the initial stages of the process to detox. While you're participating of the detoxification program completely it is not permitted to consume any food that could possibly increase the quantity of dopamine that can be produced by the body.

When an individual has finished the process of detoxification the ideal situation is they'll be more centered, balanced and less susceptible to the numerous dopamine-related triggers they feel. It is due to the fact that they be free from the drug which caused them to be experiencing these signs. However it's not possible for someone to undergo a complete dopamine detox where they can effectively prevent all dopamine-related activation within the brain. It is due to the fact that dopamine an essential neurotransmitter for normal brain functioning. The method for detoxification described above isn't even possible. It is of paramount importance that you don't ignore this momentous event.

However, even when there is no exposure to specific stimulus, the body still produces the dopamine it produces on its own. This is referred to as the endogenous dopamine generation. Endogenous dopamine production is a word used to describe this procedure. The process that involves "detoxing" from dopamine might be described more precisely by "unplugging" from the outside the world and taking a small duration of time to stay away from taking medicines that have dopamine for a certain period of duration.

People who consistently implement the program will be more likely to see positive results directly as a consequence of the time and effort that they invest in implementing the plan and increases the chances that the strategy will prove success. In contrast this term "dopamine detox" is problematic because of the very nature of the phrase as a whole and therefore cannot in any sense be considered authentic from a scientific from a scientific standpoint. In a variety of distinct occasions.

Do you think an Dopamine Detox have benefits?

We've come to the conclusion that it's impossible to conduct an effective cleansing process that is thorough and comprehensive from the dopamine naturally produced within the human body. Our research findings has led us to the conclusion.

However taking the decision to get rid of certain obsessions and break connections with them could be beneficial to the health of one's self. One of the benefits is the chance to improve concentration and mental acuity. It is among the benefits that could be reaped.

Dopamine is one of the neurotransmitters, which is known to be a great way of diverting focus, making it harder for certain people to reach their goals. This is the reason why people tend to scroll endlessly on social media and binge-watching their favourite television shows as well as actions that result in an over number of specific feel-good behavior. Also, it is the reason that causes individuals to participate in activities which result in an excess of specific feel-good behavior. This is what also leads people to engage to perform actions that generate the most amount of good feelings, and this can be the reason why they engage in those actions.

In the wake of these unnecessary obligations that people face, they are not able to better utilize their time for things like their work or efforts to maintain their health, or the maintenance of their home as well as other pursuits. It is possible that people will are able to use more of their hands to engage in pursuits and pursuits that are important to them when they take the initiative to not get distracted by all the different activities and hobbies that are accessible to people.

Dopamine detoxification isn't physically possible, and any information proving its beneficial effects can only be derived from anecdotal reports.

The people who are able attain a higher level of success number of many advantages, if they avoid certain actions like spending long periods of time scrolling using a smartphone or other social networks. This is achievable when people stop engaging in certain actions, like having a long time scrolling through smartphones and social media sites. The people will be able to attain this aim by avoiding engaging in specific activities like spending hours in a row browsing through their phones and numerous social media sites.

Chapter 10: 9 Ways To Rejuvenate Your Body

In general, the term is often used to mean the act of adhering to an imposed diet plan or usage of special products which promise to rid the body of toxins thus improving overall health and leading to losing weight. But, it can be applied to any activity that promises that the body will be cleansed of harmful toxins.

It's a good thing since your body has everything it requires to get rid of toxins. consequently, you do not have to follow specific diets or pay an enormous amount on supplements to accomplish this. If you aren't keen to take this route then you are able to eliminate the contaminants by drinking plenty of fluids and eating nutritious meals.

The naturally occurring detoxification system that's already present within your body holds the possibility of being boosted.

The book explains some of the most frequently-repeated misconceptions regarding detoxification. It also provides nine scientifically-based ways to boost your body's natural cleansing process. It also clarifies many of the common myths regarding detoxification.

A Number of Common Misconceptions Regarding the Detoxification Process

A few people have the impression that an elimination diet will allow the body cleanse of harmful toxins. It can also assist those who are attempting to achieve the weight loss goals they have set and improve their general well-being. This isn't the reality.

It's a common practice when cleansing programmes are to use medications and food items that are believed to be detoxifying. Some examples of these chemicals as well as foods are laxatives, diuretics as well as vitamins, minerals teas, food items and drinks.

In discussions about detox diets, they often use the word "toxin" is used in a way that's not completely consistent with the definition. It is due to the fact that detox diets are designed to cleanse your body of harmful toxins. The majority of times the body is comprised of chemical compounds that pollute such as synthetic chemicals, heavy metals, as well as processed foods and are considered to have an adverse influence on the health of a person.

The majority of detox programs do not provide information on the specific toxins they are attempting to eliminate, or how they plan to remove the harmful substances. The reason for this is that the elimination of certain contaminants is the principal purpose of detox diets. This is because of the fact that most of the diets that claim to cleanse your body, do not specify either one of these things.

Additionally, there is not enough evidence to justify the usage of these diets to get rid of the toxins, or to maintain an ideal weight. The claims are not confirmed by any research. The claims are not confirmed with any research study whatsoever, in any form or manner.

Removal of the body of toxins is a complex and multi-step process that requires a number of distinct organs and system. The organs and systems that are involved include the body's skin, lungs the liver, skin, and the your digestive tract.

But, for organs to fulfill their purpose to rid the body of toxic substances in a safe manner the organs must be well-maintained. They will not be able perform their tasks until when the right time comes.

Thus, although detox diets might not accomplish any results that your body could not easily do by itself however, it is possible enhance the cleansing process the body already has when you follow a certain regimen. It's despite the fact that detox diets won't achieve anything that your body can't naturally perform.

1. Limit Alcohol

The liver produces enzymes that create the acetaldehyde that is produced as a byproduct in the process of the metabolization of alcohol. Acetaldehyde is a compound which has been linked to the possibility of developing cancer. When your liver has concluded that acetaldehyde could be poisonous substance, transforms it into a form so it turns into a molecule called acetate. This is totally harmless.

Once it's completed the task it was created, the substance is eliminated from the body to ensure that it can go on living the rest of your life.

Despite the fact that studies conducted by observation have proven that moderate to low alcohol consumption can be beneficial to cardiovascular health, studies have found that over-drinking causes a myriad of health concerns. Drinking excessively is linked to the risk of dying due to cardiovascular diseases.

Intoxication from excessive alcohol could cause serious harm to the functioning of the liver. (Cause and Effect) As as a result of your liver's reaction, the damage may manifest itself in the form of a buildup of fat, inflammation as well as scarring.

In this situation the liver becomes unable to work properly and in a position to not perform the functions essential for its functioning like removing waste and other harmful toxins from the body. The result is grave health problems. As a result, it is possible to end up with many discomforts.

In direct consequence from this as a direct result, one effective method to ensure that the detoxification process within your body is operating efficiently is to drastically cut down to, or completely abstain from the consumption of alcohol drinks. This is among the best ways to ensure that the detoxification process within your body is operating efficiently.

Specialists within the field of medicine advise women to limit the consumption of alcohol to not more than one drink a day and men are advised to limit their drinking to not more than two glasses of alcohol per every day. The recommendation is to begin drinking before so that you can reap the benefits to your heart and other organs that come from moderate to light consumption. The benefits can be derived from drinking alcohol in smaller or moderate quantities. Averaging one or two drinks of alcohol every day can bring these benefits.

Ingestion of a large amount of alcohol can reduce the ability of the liver to complete the normal functions, which includes detoxification processes. This is the case especially in the event that alcohol is consumed in a way that is similar to a binge. This is particularly the case in the event that you consume a substantial amount of drinks every day.

2. Focus on Sleep

If you wish to maintain your body's health and its natural detoxification system it uses healthy, then it is essential to make sure that you're getting sufficient rest each night and ensure that you are getting enough rest throughout the day. If you're not doing this do this, it will be difficult to keep your body as well as its natural detoxification system it uses in good health.

Your brain has the ability to remodel and regenerate itself as you're asleep in addition to rid its own of dangerous leftovers from the day. The process can take place during your sleep. The process of forming neurons is known as neurogenesis.

One of the byproducts is a protein which is called beta-amyloid which is among the causes that lead to the development of Alzheimer's Disease. Another of these byproducts is a peptide called alpha-synuclein.

If you're not getting enough rest then your body will not get enough time to complete these processes. This can lead to the accumulation of toxins which can adversely impact multiple aspects of your well-being. If you're not getting enough rest, strive to get at least 7 hours of rest each at night. If you get sufficient sleep the body will get sufficient time complete those actions.

It's been proven that not sleeping enough can have immediate as well longer-lasting negative consequences for a person's overall health. The negative consequences may be temporary and lasting. They can result in the increase of stress levels and anxiety, and also the high blood pressure as well as heart disease, type 2 diabetes and weight gain.

For those who want to keep the healthiest lifestyle it is essential to set a goal to make sure that people get enough sleep every the night (seven to 9 hours).

If you are having trouble sleeping or remaining in bed at night, make modifications to your life like adhering to your sleep routine and restricting your exposure to blue lights (emitted through mobile devices as well as computer screens) throughout the days before bedtime could help improve the quality of sleep that you are able to get. If you're having difficulty sleeping or staying asleep during the time of night, making changes to your life can aid in improving the quality of sleep that you receive. Changes in this kind of lifestyle can aid in improving sleeping quality enjoyed by the person.

3. Drink More Water

The benefits of drinking water is a great way to ease your dry mouth and sore throat The benefits from drinking it go beyond the obvious. The body's temperature stays stable and joints are kept well-lubricated, digestion is improved and digestion of nutrients is improved as well as your body gets cleansed as a result of elimination of waste material in your system.

Cells are always in need of being repaired to ensure that they remain functioning properly and breakdown the nutrients in order that your body uses them as fuel. The repair process must be carried out to allow your cells to function properly. It is vital your cells within your body continue functioning properly and process nutrients.

However the process results in the creation of waste products that is a form of carbon dioxide and urea. Both are thought to be waste materials. If you allow either of these substances build up at a level that is harmful to the blood over a prolonged duration then you place your health at risk.

They are carried through the water system and allow it to be possible for them to get rid of much more effectively through breath, urine and sweat. (Citation required) As a result being the case, it's essential to detoxification processes to ensure the right amount of water is available in all instances.

It is suggested that men drink the equivalent of 125 in ounces (3.7 Liters) of drinking water every day whereas women need to consume 91 ounces. The recommended amount of water is recommended to be consumed every day by males is the equivalent of 125 pounds (3.7 Liters) (2.7 Liters). It's possible that the amount of specific nutrient you need can be greater or less in your case based on what kind of food are consumed, the surroundings that you live in and the degree of physical exercise that you engage in.

4. Decrease the Quantity of Sugar and Processed Foods That You Consume Daily.

Foods that are processed and sugar that has been processed appear as being the major cause of current health conditions that harm the health of people everywhere.

There's a connection between eating foods which are processed as well as high in sugar, and a higher likelihood of becoming obese along with other chronic diseases like cancer, diabetes or heart problems. The risk of obesity is high for these diseases.

These conditions cause harm to organs like kidneys and the liver that are essential for our body's daily elimination process but may be affected by the conditions. In the aftermath of this, it'll become more difficult for your body to be able to get rid of the toxins it has in its own.

In particular, there's evidence of an association between the consumption of excessive amounts of alcohol that is sugary and creation of a condition referred to as fat liver. It has been demonstrated to cause harm on the functions that the liver performs. Drinking a lot of sweet drinks has been associated with this problem.

Cut down on the quantity of junk foods you consume in order to maintain your body's detoxification system in top condition. This can be achieved by limiting the quantity of food that is junk.

One way of reducing the intake of unhealthy foods is to ensure the current supply of the food items at retail stores, as that's one method to achieve this. If you don't own it at home and you're not tempted to eat it. That means that you will not have to be concerned about this aspect of the matter.

Consumption can be cut down to a healthier level by selecting healthier options for eating including veggies and fruits, as opposed to those with fewer nutrients like junk food. A change in eating habits could help lower total caloric consumption. This could lead to less consumption in general.

5. Include in Your Diet a Variety of Foods That Are Known to Contain a High Amount of Antioxidants

Antioxidants protect the cells of your body from dangers caused by free radicals, as well as other harmful chemical compounds. Due to their ability to be unstable this chemical has the ability to cause damage. An issue resulted from an unusually high amount of free radicals is known as an oxidative stress. The condition could have adverse impacts on the health of a person.

The body can be capable of producing these substances in its own way due to natural processes like digestion, and various cellular processes. Additionally, other natural processes help in the process. However there are lots of causes that could be responsible for the development in excess free radicals. A few of them are smoking cigarettes, eating a poor diet, drinking a large quantity of alcohol and getting exposed to pollutant.

These proteins have been connected to various ailments, like dementia, heart disease asthma, liver disease as well as certain types of cancer due to the fact they can cause damages to the cells of the body. Since they are those responsible for causing the harm which is for.

Eating a diet packed with antioxidants could aid the body in fighting acidity that's caused due to an over-abundance of free radicals, as well as other contaminants that increase the chance of developing illness. This is accomplished through consuming a food which is rich in antioxidants. This can be done by eating food items that are rich in antioxidants, and providing your body the nutrients it needs.

The most effective way to be sure you're receiving enough antioxidants from your food is to take these from foods you consume rather than tablets. Tablets when taken in adequate quantities, could make it more likely of developing certain illnesses. Incorporating antioxidants into the foods which you consume is the most efficient method to ensure that you're getting adequate antioxidants into your diet.

Antioxidants can be found in a array of forms. The most popular of them include vitamin A, C, and E along with selenium, as well as lycopene, Zeaxanthin, and lutein. Another example of this is the color called zeaxanthin.

The highest amounts of antioxidants are present in drinks and foods like berries, fruits chocolate, nuts, vegetables spice, beverages such as green tea and coffee. Nuts, fruits, berries as well as chocolate have significant amounts of antioxidants. Coffee and green tea are just two of the food items and drinks that are able to contain an abundance of antioxidants.

6. Eat a diet full of foods containing prebiotics. Make sure you keep it up to date.

A healthy gut is vital to the general health of your detoxification process, and it will aid to achieve your goal. The digestive system as well as the remainder of your body are safeguarded against harmful toxins through the process of detoxification and excreta which is located in the intestinal cell tract. The lymphatic system in your body is home to this specific procedure (such as chemical substances).

A particular type of fiber called prebiotics serves as a source of nutrition for beneficial bacteria within the digestive tract, referred to as probiotics. Probiotics reside within the stomach. Prebiotics are the initial stage towards maintaining a healthy digestive tract. If you provide the beneficial bacteria you have prebiotics to take in, the bacterial population of your body will have the ability to create chemicals that are known as short-chain fatty acid. These chemicals are good for the health of your body. If you feed your beneficial bacteria by introducing prebiotics to them, they'll be in a position to create the wonderful nutrients you need to your body that will benefit your overall well-being.

If you take antibiotics, do not practice good dental hygiene or eat meals that aren't high-quality It is likely that the beneficial bacteria living inside your stomach to get off-balance with the harmful bacteria living in the intestines of your. It can happen when you consume food items that are not of high-quality.

The unfavourable change to the microorganisms within your body can trigger your immune and detoxification system to weaken This could increase the risk of developing disease and inflammation.

Ingestion of meals high in prebiotics may help keep an immune system that is healthy and an effective detoxification system functioning properly within the body. Prebiotics are present in various food items. Artichokes, tomatoes, bananas as well as asparagus, garlic, onions, and oats are among products that offer the highest amount of prebiotics present in foods. Other great sources of prebiotics include garlic, onions and onions. Onions, garlic as well as onions are just three other ingredients that provide a good amount of this substance.

7. Cut down on the amount of sodium you consume into your body on regular on a regular basis.

A few people might find cleansing aids by releasing excess water their bodies has been holding onto however, others may not notice this advantage.

If you suffer from a condition that impacts your kidneys or liver, or you aren't drinking enough water or eat a large quantity of salt could result in your body retaining the excess amount of fluid. It can occur even when you drink a lot of water. This condition if you aren't drinking sufficient water intake on a regular routine. This can be particularly true when your meals contain substantial amounts of salt, and you get the salt into your system.

Many people experience abdominal constipated due to the accumulation of fluids in their body. This can make it hard to put on clothes. This could be particularly problematic in pregnant women. If you realize that you're taking in the wrong amount of salt, it is possible to detox your body to rid yourself of excess water weight has accumulated.

This may sound contradictory yet increasing the amount of water you drink is among the best strategies for lower the amount of water weight caused by eating excessive amounts of salt. The weight gain occurs because the body is retaining more water than it has to. The weight gain is a consequence of the body's retention of an excessive amount of water in comparison to the amount it ought to.

It is because of the nature of your body to create an antidiuretic hormonal hormone that prevents the need to go through a urination when you consume excess amounts of salt, while drinking a small quantity of water. This hormone prevents the need to go through urinate. This is because you'll hold greater amounts of water than normal for your body (and consequently cleansing).

When you drink a lot of water, the body's metabolism will decrease the hormone responsible for reducing diuresis as well as produce more urine, which can result in the elimination of more waste and water substances. It is due to diuresis being the procedure that your body uses to eliminate the waste as well as excess water. It is because of the reality that the body can produce less of the hormone which inhibits the process of urination.

The increase in the quantity of foods you eat that are rich in potassium could be helpful since it assists in reduce some of the negative effects that salt can have on your body. The effects of salt include the retention of water, muscle cramps and elevated blood pressure. The squash, potatoes and kidney beans, as well as spinach, and bananas are a few examples of food items which have high amount of potassium per serving.

8. Do some exercises

What ever you weigh, participating with regular exercise can reduce chances of developing many ailments and illnesses, such as type 2 heart disease, diabetes high blood pressure and certain malignancies. It is the same regardless of whether you're overweight. There is no distinction whether you smoke cigarettes or not, this is the norm. This is the case regardless of whether the person is involved physically in any kind of sport.

Although there are numerous distinct mechanisms that account for the positive effects that exercise brings to the body, one of the procedures that are responsible for significant reductions in inflammation is among the most significant of these procedures.

Although inflammation is essential to heal injuries and recovery of infections, chronic inflammation causes your body's systems to be more vulnerable to disease and weakens them all over.

The exercise routine can aid in ensuring that your body's system, especially the detoxification system. This helps it work better, and protect you from disease. This happens because exercise reduces inflammation present within the body.

It is suggested that you engage for at least 75-150 minutes per week high-intensity exercise, like running or engaging in moderate intensity physical exercise, like brisk walking, at least 150-300 minutes per week, in order to ensure a healthy life style.

9. Additional Useful Hints, Guidelines, and Counsel Regarding the Detoxification Process

While there's not enough evidence to justify the usage of detox diets in the hopes of eliminating toxic substances from your body specific dietary modifications as well as lifestyle changes can assist to reduce the amount of toxins within your body, and also increasing the effectiveness of your body's natural detoxification system. The majority of sulfur comes in the food you eat as it contains plenty of sulfur. Foods that are high in sulfur such as broccoli, onions, as well as garlic, could aid in the removal of heavy metals from your body easier. This could be so because broccoli, onions, as well as garlic, are all foods that are sulfur-rich. The heavy metals are symbolized as cadmium for one instance.

Think about injecting chlorella into your system. Chlorella is a kind of algae, which according to studies carried out on animals, offers numerous benefits to the nutrition of people and the ability to aid the body in the elimination of harmful elements like heavy metals. The benefits of chlorella can stem by the fact that chlorella is a type of algae.

The taste of food items can be improved with the use of the herb cilantro. Toxins like lead, as well as other heavy metals, as well as to pollutants, such as pesticides and phthalates, can be eliminated from your body in a much more efficient manner when you consume cilantro.

It is important to support the glutathione. Glutathione is a powerful antioxidant that plays a significant role in detoxification and made by the body, is among the key players in the process. The antioxidant glutathione plays a crucial important to the process. Consuming food items that are high in sulfur, such as broccoli, eggs, as well as garlic, may aid in the improvement of the performance of glutathione within the body. It is due to glutathione being an antioxidant, which protects cells from injury.

Make the switch to cleaning solutions made from natural materials instead of the ones typically utilized. If you wash your home using substances that are natural instead of conventional cleaning products it will lessen your exposure to hazardous chemicals that are in the environment. Natural cleaners include vinegar, baking soda as well as essential oils. Vinegar and baking soda are just two examples of things that can be considered to be natural cleaners.

When it comes to your body-care routine, opt for organic items whenever possible. Using organic alternatives to cosmetics such as deodorants, cosmetics and shampoos and moisturizers can aid in reducing the quantity of toxic chemicals you're exposed. This means reducing the number of toxic chemicals found in your items. This could benefit your health over the long term.

Although a lot of them appear to be beneficial However, a majority are only confirmed through experiments conducted in animals. However, it is true that a lot of the impacts are positive in nature. In direct consequence of this, these results require confirmation with research done on individuals within their environments.

Chapter 11: The Use Of Mindfulness As A Tool For Overcoming The Habit Of Procrastination

While understanding these mind games can help us understand our habit of never putting off tasks but there's no assurance that we'll succeed in breaking the pattern even after having this knowledge. There is a good chance that one method that has proven to be the most successful to conquer procrastination is beat it. You can train your brain to react differently when you are confronted by a job or task which you do not find appealing. How? Mindfulness. Don't do let the popularity of the term deter people from practicing mindfulness. the only thing you need to do to get started on the path of mindfulness is to allow you to be fully conscious of all that occurs around you as well as within your own body at any time. It is a simple process of being aware and interested about your sensations in response to an the cause (for instance you're hungry, and would rather not send this email, and being close to that person makes me anxious) This is the most important step in reducing anxiety as well as breaking bad habit patterns like procrastination. As an instance, I'm hungry. I'm not going to write this email, and proximity to this person can make me feel anxious. For a couple of examples: I'm hungry, I'm afraid to write this email And being in the presence causes me to be anxious.

It is paradoxically efficient because it involves us directly with the process of reward in order help us move away from the habit of reward-based thinking. This is because Mindfulness acts as the creator of reward. when you are thinking about food and you decide to eat then your stomach transmits an euphoric signal to your brain that informs that it about what you had eaten and the location you ate the food.

On contrary, could be linked to the very same thing which causes stress and worry at the beginning. It's designed to work as a loop that facilitates the development of habitual behavior." The only distinction is that it operates opposite to the other way around.

A task or project which needs to be completed is a prime example of an event trigger that could be utilized. As avoiding it leads to more satisfaction overall the majority of people choose to avoid the trigger. The relief and consolation that you feel as a result being able to not do it will pay off even though the sensations will not last very time. " Since the avoided activity causes the discomfort to disappear instantly because it causes discomfort. the avoidance process gives an immediate feeling of calm which acts as a trigger to the continuance of delay.

The author continues, "There is a great deal of scientific research suggesting that mindfulness is very effective at attacking these habit loops." As a result, we have the ability to accomplish two things. First they can recognize how unrewarding our old behaviour is. This is one of the advantages. For a different perspective simply start to realize how frightened feeling, terrified, and overwhelmed it is to put off doing something. You shouldn't berate or blame yourself for this; instead begin to be aware of it and accepting the fact that it is a reality. Sooner or later, you will realize that it's not only negative, but is also quite unpleasant in the long run to voluntarily submit to feelings such as these. You soon will understand.

The other thing it can do is provides a more effective alternative to what was offered previously. It was this second aspect it could do. Involve yourself in the mind of an attentive person through practicing one of its main features of being inquisitive. Engaging in your feelings as well as your emotions and bodily sensations could result in situations which are not as enjoyable the moment you're engaged and engaged with these parts of your life. "We actually have the capability of teaching ourselves to substitute enquiry for procrastination as a learning strategy. We are able, through the practice of mindfulness, to see the [positive] results of really completing our assignment."

Give it a shot for a single time to check to see if you are able to finish your task sooner than you anticipated (or in time and if it's something option for you and we don't care about it!) Don't allow the weight of it to continue to burden your shoulders. There is a good chance that you will experience the following: "You are successful in completing the task at hand, you put your phone on silent, and you focus on one activity at a time rather than trying to juggle many things at once. After that, all you need to do is take note of how incredible it feels when you finally finish it. Mindfulness practice can help our brain get the information it needs whether we are putting off productive activities or actively engaged in productive action."

If you are the next person to notice yourself holding off on the next task, pay notice of how you're thinking about the task (does it cause you to feel uncomfortable, sweaty, annoyed or even overwhelmed?). This can help you decide which option to make it a priority to get the task accomplished. Once you've had time to give the idea some thought, consider the task a shot and then see if it's possible to notice a change regarding how the longer-lasting and more gratifying feeling can make you feel (accomplished as well as proud and more relaxed). The likelihood is that it won't take long before you begin to develop an addiction to this brand new and healthy cycle of habit.

The Step-by-Step Guide to Overcoming Your Dependence on Dopamine and Getting Your Life Back on Track

Given the strong feelings that come with dopamine, it won't require a long time for a person to fall in love with the drug. The findings have been taken as evidence in support of an idea that neurotransmitter dopamine is itself addicted, and not the drugs or actions that cause the increase in its levels.

In order to answer the question of whether or not it's feasible to be addicted to dopamine you need to first understand the functions of dopamine inside the brain, as well as the characteristics of addiction. Then, you will be able determine

There is a possibility of becoming dependent on dopamine.

A deficiency of dopamine or an excess of it are likely to cause a significant negative effect on one's overall well-being.

If you are looking for an dopamine addiction It isn't evident if someone is addicted to the chemical dopamine by itself, or by the action or behaviour which results in the creation of dopamine. It is likely that one might be dependent on both. It is a subject that is in the process of being debated by several groups at present. The latter view is supported by the overwhelming majority of scientists in the science field. It is crucial to gain an understanding of the causes of addiction as well as the function that dopamine plays in the functioning of the brain to determine the cause of the issue.

What exactly is it in this? What makes it so captivating?

Dopamine can make people feel great. The reason for this is that it creates within us the sensation of being acknowledged by some manner to participate in the activity we decide to engage in. This motivates us to engage in this behavior often that is what we want to result. Furthermore, they encourage us to fulfill the basic requirements for existence, like eating foods. The reward and incentive program is a great option, if no one of us suffers from an addiction like the heroin addiction. If we do suffer from addictions like that, this program is not working. If we get the goals we set We are more likely to pursue what we desire, and once we achieve what we desire then we get a feeling of satisfaction.

If there is a sense of anticipation of the reward to receive then the body begins the release of dopamine. The sensation of having been recognized is briefly replaced by enthusiasm when we are presented with the reward, but it soon fades away. It is our goal to recreate the feeling in our own lives. Is this implying that we are aiming for dopamine as the ultimate aim we're looking to achieve? Yes, however according to a scientific viewpoint that is not the case. What we're searching for is the chemicals or actions that possess the capacity to deliver the dopamine we need. Dopamine isn't the only thing in itself that causes the addiction, but rather it's the result of the additional substances and behaviours.

Dopamine levels are low, you might suffer from these symptoms:

In the absence of dopamine the body would find it physically impossible to live.

If you didn't have the hormone, there's absolutely nothing you can do within this universe. If you were in that situation there is no way you would even be capable of moving even a centimeter in either direction. If you're in possession of dopamine but not enough It is possible for you to be suffering from one or more of the various diseases that can be linked to being deficient in dopamine.

* Parkinson's Disease

* Depression

* Alzheimer's Disease

* Social Phobia

* Social Anxiety Disorder * Social Phobic Disorder

What are Some of the Repercussions That Come With Having an Excessive Amount?

Based on the results of a variety of studies, having high levels of dopamine levels in the brain has been associated with mental illnesses including schizophrenia. It's a complex disorder that impacts a variety of specific brain areas and is impaired in some way due to schizophrenia. The problem is that this high concentration of dopamine isn't due to addiction to dopamine, or a desire for it, but rather it's the result of excessive production of dopamine by the body. Dopamine is released in overflow within your body due to the condition called hyperdopaminergic excessive.

Is There a Connection Between Being Addicted to Dopamine and Developing Other Disorders, Both Physical and Mental?

There's a link between issues with the dopamine system as well as a variety of illnesses, both mental as well as physical.

Could this mean that the dopamine system is the main cause of the disorders? In the moment, only an insignificant amount of data is available. Dopamine's connection to addiction is complex with the particulars of how it manifests vary based on the condition that is causing it. It is possible that the diseases are triggered through other causes as well, so the malfunction in the dopamine structure is just one of the signs of the disorder. The majority of the diseases and conditions listed below are related to malfunctions of the dopamine system and consequently they fall as such.

Major depression as well as dependence dopamine can be a sign of this disorder.

Based on the results from several studies the evidence suggests a clear link between dopamine levels and symptoms of depression. In contrast when you are suffering from depressive symptoms, then dopamine likely to not be the sole neurotransmitter at work with your particular condition. Because of dopamine's effects some people are more likely to suffer from depression more than others. It is so in relation with other individuals. Your particular biochemical makeup determines the role of dopamine in the therapy approach you choose in treating your depression. Depression, and its associated shifts in dopamine levels tend to be linked with the formation of addiction. (Case in Point: (Case in Point: (Case in Point:) Antidepressants acting as dopamine-receptor antagonists such as bupropion can be effective therapeutic options for many mental health disorders, like addiction and depression. This is because the relationship between dopamine and depression can be vital to treating a wide range of illnesses, such as addiction. (Cause and Effect)

Bipolar illness and dopamine are closely linked.

The hypothesis that bipolar is based on dopamine disease suggests that dopamine is an essential role in both manic and depressed phases of the disorder however, the theory is considered as an old idea by the scientific community. When a person is in mania that dopamine released to the brain is at an all-time high. If someone is depressed the levels of dopamine are significantly lower than they would be. Also, it is important to recognize that as the manic stage develops as it progresses, the dopamine receptors decreases and eventually cause depression. The manic stage is accompanied by a return back to the depression phase as receptors get more sensitive in this phase. The phase of depressing is marked by decreased transmission that are later followed by a return back to the mania.

ADHD And Dopamine

Use of stimulants is the most common type of treatment that children receive when they are diagnosed as having ADHD. One of the main worries that parents face is the possibility that their child's treatment for ADHD as well as the dopamine-related consequences that come to it could lead their child to become addicted to substances later on. It is among the main concerns parents are faced with. But, it's an established fact that when children are treated for ADHD through this way and are treated in this manner, they not only will be less susceptible to getting into trouble with drugs and also less of a tendency to smoke cigarettes. Dopamine deficiency in the context of ADHD is a common problem. (ADHD) is the current subject of studies that aim to discover solutions that are secure and efficient and focuses on treatment for children.

Dopamine And Parkinson's

Dopamine insufficiency has been linked to difficulties with mental state, movements as well as memory. These all can contribute to the wide array of signs and symptoms associated in Parkinson's. The disease of Parkinson's is characterised by many manifestations. A decline in the dopamine receptor system common to Parkinson's condition is the primary basis of the failure. Due to this decline, the quantity of dopamine receptors present in the brain is reduced. In turn, this results in a decrease in the frequency and intensity of dopamine-related impulses. This can lead to issues with memory. The quantity of neurons in the brain that are responsible for producing dopamine decreases steadily with age and results in an ongoing decline in the levels of dopamine. Researchers are dedicating a large amount of their time and effort to the study of the relationship between Parkinson's disease and dopamine, with the intention to develop treatments to treat the dysfunction of dopamine caused by Parkinson's disease. Dopamine's challenges generated in Parkinson's diseases are the focus of this study and aims to discover feasible therapeutic alternatives. This research was funded with the help of National Institutes of Health (NIH).

Dopamine And Schizophrenia

The hypothesis that schizophrenia is caused by dopamine claims that schizophrenia is a condition which develops because of an excessive quantity of dopamine that is present within the brain. The research initiated by academics who began studying the link between schizophrenia and dopamine and this led to a discussion among scientists. It led to the creation of this theory and grew due to the fact that neuroleptic medications are able to reduce dopamine and proved to be effective in treating schizophrenia. However, drugs that increased dopamine make the illness more severe. It was concluded that neuroleptic medications are the ones that decrease dopamine and can be responsible for this. Because of this research, scientists recognized that "neuro" is the root of the neuroleptic drugs, which have been proven to reduce dopamine levels. In contrast it is believed that the link with schizophrenia as well as dopamine have not been fully explored yet. It is due to the fact that people who are healthy don't develop symptoms of schizophrenia when receiving high doses of dopamine. people with schizophrenia are not all can benefit from treatment using neuroleptic drugs.

Dopamine can be released into the brain in response to of certain actions.

In spite of the fact that it was said previously, the issue of whether dopamine-related dysfunctions could cause dependency on dopamine remains not resolved. Dopamine deficiencies can result in mental as well as physical ailments like the one mentioned earlier. Researchers who study dopamine in the area of science have an opinion that, when people talk about their addiction to dopamine, they are really saying is that they're enthralled by actions that cause the body to produce dopamine. For an appreciation of this concept it is first necessary be aware of several of the more common actions that trigger the creation of dopamine. Then, you will get more understanding of this argument.

Porn And Dopamine

Dopamine releases into the system every time pornography is seen as well, and this is amplified when watching porn regularly. There is a possibility of experiencing an euphoria just when you realize that you're about to view some explicit material. It's likely to be fun watching it, however the amount of satisfaction you'll experience from it will not be able to match the anticipation that you'll feel prior to the event.

Dopamine levels in our bodies gradually diminish as more people are exposed to pornographic films. This is why dopamine-related transmissions diminish in the process of. In the event of this then it's likely that you'll be tempted to be more prone to pornographic entertainment and this will result in an endless pattern of addiction which gets more and more serious as time passes until the point at when you are treated.

Dopamine And Sex

A variety of studies show the connection between dopamine and sexual activity. Researchers believe that the evolution process that created the dopamine system was designed to ensure that animals could be able to live.

The reason for this idea. The prehistoric period required individuals to engage with sexual activity so as to ensure the survival of their species. This suggests that there's an immediate connection between the dopamine system when you engage in sexual relations with someone else. When you experience extreme desire for sexual activities until the point where others aspects of your daily life are put at risk, then you could be suffering from a disorder which is in danger of turning into addicted. If you go through therapy and treatment, you'll be taught ways to curb these cravings completely. If you can attain this goal and live a an enviable and secure life are greatly enhanced.

Dopamine and cocaine are also in the process.

Dopamine as well as cocaine comprise two chemical compounds that often occur when they are in conjunction with each other. When you drink cocaine, the brain reacts to release dopamine. This can cause you to feel joyous (at at least for a short time).

This is due to the substance in itself. It is true that it is so powerful that you wish to repeat the experience whenever it's physically possible to do it. Your dopamine system is likely to alter over time and with it increase the amount of dopamine receptors in use for the cocaine reward as well as other kinds of pleasures and different types of dopamine signals will decline. Dopamine receptors play a role in the processing of satisfactions and rewards. That is the higher your dose of cocaine more, the lower amount of dopamine that your brain creates contrary to the time the first time you started using the drug.

This is referred to as the dose-response relation. Once you have stopped having the medication it is possible to notice that you feel a strong desire for the drug, but the enjoyment that you experience from it could be less intense. The evidence suggests that a malfunction in the dopamine pathway caused by cocaine can alter the chemical makeup of your brain in time. If you've at this point It is crucial for you to engage in treatment to treat the problem and bring your dopamine level back to an equilibrium.

Marijuana And Dopamine

Marijuana is a substances that are used frequently and consumed throughout America. United States. The question that needs to be addressed now is what exactly is the link between marijuana and dopamine? It's been proven that using marijuana over an extended period can have a negative impact on the reward system based on dopamine. (Citation required) The amounts of dopamine created through all illegal substances have effects on the nucleus of accumbens located in the brain active in the anticipation of reward in the dopamine brain. The effects of marijuana could alter the dopamine receptors in ways that prolongation of usage of other substances, and even dependence on those substances, can cause.

Dopamine and Alcohol's Influence on One Another

With regard to dopamine and alcohol, reactions in the dopamine pathway to reward non-drug substances decrease when addiction develops similar fashion to how they do in other substances and behaviors. The mesolimbic area is the place in which this process plays through. Loss of control over behavior results from an interruption in the second dopamine pathway that acts as an inhibitory control. The disruption in the system causes it to be unstable. The amount of dopamine released will decrease because of changes occurring within the dopamine system over your life. Because of this, you'll need more alcohol to achieve that same degree in "feel good" that you experienced when drinking.

Combating addiction can be won, and is a battle that could be taken on.

But what we're conscious of is that healthy people have a dopamine system which operates normally and is stable. Even though the mechanisms behind dopamine, addiction, as well as other conditions are not entirely understood, this is what happens. There is no distinction between whether you're dependent on dopamine or the process that produces dopamine. The battle against addiction is winnable, like it was in the past for millions of previous people.

How to End Your Addiction to Dopamine and Regain Control of Your Life

There's no magic remedy or a method that will treat dopamine dependent effectively in everyone struggling with the condition. But there's a myriad of different things you could take to increase your odds of success and put yourself in a higher situation. Here is a listing of various strategies which can be employed by you to beat the addiction you are fighting.

Chapter 12: What Is Dopamine?

Dopamine is an example of a synapse. Responsible for transferring signals to the neurons of the brain Dopamine is often referred to as an artificial courier. It is a significant area of our body, and directly affects the central sensorimotor system.

Qualities

Dopamine is often referred in the context of being the "delight substance," this is not the case, since dopamine does not bring joy. But it can provide feelings of happiness by bringing joyous vibes with certain practices.

"It's a vibe decent substance," claims Tanya J. Peterson, NCC, DAIS, a psychologist and instructor. "It's essential for our award community, and when our mind produces dopamine in light of what we do, we feel better and need to accomplish a greater amount of whatever it is that is causing us to feel so intellectually amazing. That, thus, prompts considerably more dopamine creation."

Dopamine also plays a role in our instinctual reactions. When confronted with a risk, real or imagined that the thought-provoking sensor system (SNS) begins to activate and triggers the release of catecholamines and dopamine to help the body react to the stress.

Dopamine can be produced in a number of locations in the cerebrum states James Giordano, MD, MPhil, professor of nerve system biology and natural chemical chemistry in the Georgetown University Medical Center, which includes the substantia nigra ventral tegmental zone and the pituitary organ as well as in the pathways that connect to the nerve centers.

The Role of Dopamine in the Body

Dopamine directly affects a variety of cognitive, neurological and social functions within the body, according to Dr. Giordano. These include:

- Movement

Reward and reinforcement

Feelings, thoughts and thoughts

- Arousal

- Regulating specific organs and chemicals

Dopamine can affect everything in our thinking and behave to the way we act and remember. Dopamine affects us all uniquely, and a shift in the levels of dopamine is hard to determine, but it is a clear sign that dopamine affects the health of our emotional and physical wellbeing.

A high or excessive amount of dopamine could cause a variety of problems.

Dopamine deficiency may experience a variety of signs, like

The loss of equilibrium

- Weight changes

- Muscle cramps

Energy consumption is low.

- Anxiety

- - Mood changes

Drive - Low sex

- Constipation

- Tremors

- Difficulty dozing

- Hallucinations

Although significant levels of dopamine will increase your fixation of energy, focus, sexual drive and capacity to concentrate however, it also can trigger aggressive, violent behavior and produce side effects such as anxiety, restlessness, and tension.

Wellbeing and Mental Health Disorders

When you are suffering from a dopamine problem there could be an increase in your neurocognitive capacity that are related to your attention span, memory and thinking skills.

Similar to the serotonin synapse, that manages the temperament of people, dopamine can be associated to a myriad of mental disorders. Dopamine receptors which aren't normally working play an important role in a variety of health as well-being problems.

Parkinson's Disease

Dopamine levels are reduced and can be seen in certain neurodegenerative diseases including Parkinson's illness that affects nerve cells, and the ones accountable for the delivering and delivery of dopamine have passed on to the next generation to the next generation, Professor. Giordano clarifies.

Inability to focus consistently disorder (ADHD)

Research has shown the presence of dopamine-related disorders for those who suffer from ADHD and are linked to signs of impulsivity and carelessness. Individuals who suffer from ADHD could be afflicted by prize and motivational issues, which render them unable to modify their behavior to adapt to the changing requirements of awards.

Schizophrenia

Schizophrenia is a result of changes to the brain dopamine receptors just like dopamine signaling pathways.

Antipsychotic medicines can be used as an antagonist to dopamine aiding a small number of patients suffering from schizophrenia.

Substance Use Disorder and Addiction

Dopamine-triggered reactions are triggered by certain actions such as drinking alcohol gambling, or drinking alcohol, may trigger dependency. What is the reason why certain people struggle with dependency beyond the fact that it might have in common using previous-generation dopamine-related circuits?

Significant Depressive Disorder (MDD)

MDD is among the most widely-known mental health disorders. Dopamine insufficiency could cause anhedonia, a lack of ability to experience joy and happy, a common consequence of MDD.

Chapter 13: Want To Eat Greasy Or Possibly Sweet Food Sources

A decrease in pleasure and longing with different activities

- Charisma changes

In these instances the doctor. Giordano explains the patients could be treated using energizers to increase the effects of dopamine available on its receptors as well as increase dopamine-interceded effects to reduce the signs and adverse consequences.

If you're experiencing negative consequences of an physical or emotional wellbeing issue due to of an irregularity in dopamine Treatment will be based on the cause. If you're experiencing specific symptoms, it is important consult your primary care doctor regarding your habits of eating, lifestyle, as well as your medical history, to make a decision on which of the next best treatments is appropriate for you.

Normal Ways to Balance Dopamine Levels

Dopamine levels are difficult to detect since they occur in the brain. However there are methods of changing your levels of dopamine with no prescribing. The best method of changing your dopamine levels is to focus on the most beneficial patterns of dopamine.

If you're a participant in certain dopamine-producing activities like sexual sex, innovative betting or sex it's likely that you'll require regular breaks, but if you're struggling to concentrate and feeling dismotivated or exhausted, then you'll have to increase the amount of dopamine you're creating.

Burn-through Nutritious Foods

"The supplements in specific food varieties travel to the cerebrum and add to dopamine creation," claims Peterson. The consumption of a variety of fruits and vegetables in the soil, especially bananas, may increase the production of dopamine.

Peterson also suggests protein such as fish, lean meats beans, legumes, and plants-based proteins, as well as foods that are rich in omega-3 unsaturated fats such as mackerel and salmon ground flaxseeds and pecans, chia seeds and.

Exercise Regularly

Walking for a few minutes or rehearsing yoga exercises, moving around your kitchen, or even doing a home workout helps in the delivery of sound dopamine levels. Training can also help develop relaxation propensities that keeps the dopamine levels in check.

"Do any actual work that you appreciate. Constraining yourself to accomplish something you disdain only for exercise might bring actual advantages, however for the full psychological well-being advantage related with dopamine specifically, pick development that you find pleasurable," Says Peterson.

Praise the Small Moments

"Accomplishing something little that you appreciate and intentionally interfacing that demonstration to an achievement or something awesome you notice lets your mind know that something incredible is going on and that no doubt about it," Peterson says. Peterson.

It could be simple as noticing blossoms in the garden and being aware of your primary melody, smell of espresso beans or blowing bubbles. The dopamine release will increase production, Peterson states the process, and provide you with the emotional health aid that continues to improve.

A Word From Verywell

If you're concerned regarding your levels of dopamine take care to talk with your doctor. Because dopamine is a important role in the cerebrum and body and brain, you must address the issue. Just be aware that lots of people have dopamine levels that are not balanced however, these levels can be easily altered.

Most effective way to avoid distraction Focus: Tips for Practical Use to Improve your focus

Finding a way to ensure that you don't be diverted from your work is a crucial goal to achieve. The majority of the time, you are in your office ready to finally end, finish your work. "Alright, let's do this," you think to yourself. Then you go the options of Word or Google Drive and open up an archive. There is some discussion about the best way to go about it however, what happens right away?

You write a few phrases, but you aren't able to keep the right track. At that point you decide, "Perhaps I should awaken myself with something fun." You log onto Facebook. you're gone for 20 minutes. At that point there's an hour spent inattention to a small collection of YouTube footage. In a flash, the noon hour has arrived and a significant portion of the day has passed. longer.

If it sounds like a natural thing, remember that it's not necessary to be this way. It is best to focus at the end of this post for tips on how not to be distracted.

However, before we move on to the suggestions take note of the fact that staying clear from interruptions can be a challenge. It's tough to remain focus when you have to be working for a lengthy period of time however, some people can manage it. It's a matter of why they are doing it and not you?

Additionally, it is likely that you never taught to find your center. When you were in school, the teacher likely was worried when your mind wandered and you sat staring out of the window. However, it wasn't solved by teaching you how to center. the idea was that everything would be able to fall back to the right its proper place. It's just absurd, especially given the current frenzied world.

In the end, as everyone is being plugged into their phones and devices, you have to figure out ways to maintain your focus. This is exactly what these suggestions are designed for, to help you at be able to stay focused and focused on what you're supposed to accomplish.

Remember Your Vision and Goals

Get a good foundation for your focus as you discover ways to keep your focus free of interruption. This means figuring out exactly what you must be focused on regardless of. Are you preparing for a big event at work a next week that you must prepare for? Are you thinking concerning learning to play guitar, and have to focus on it for a full hour each day as you work?

Deciding what the ultimate goal is, will help you in finding out the best way to focus. Understanding the reasons we must keep our focus on the goal can help in tackling those monotonous and arduous steps of reaching our goals. This is when the point that our concentration is really tested, and it's needed.

Lessen the Chaos of Your Day

In the event that you're assigned 20 projects that have to complete every day, what's the best way to you think your capacity for the center is?

It's impossible to imagine doing these complex things if you're not able to contemplate focusing. The trick is to keep things down to basics, as you try to determine how you can avoid getting distracted.

Concentrate on doing 3 significant projects per day but not quite that. That's all it takes to get moving towards the goals you set for yourself. Slower is superior to giving up early due to having did something that was that was too much, quickly. It's also healthier for your psychological well-being since you'll continue to see yourself moving forward without becoming stressed.

Do Those Tasks quickly

For you to make sure that you can get the two to three errands completed, it is essential to start them early so that you can focus to the task without feeling exhausted. So, when you wake up at night, you're planning how to complete them.

It's a bit extreme, and waiting to tackle these things later will allow interruptions that can be overwhelming. The interruptions can come in the form of alarming messages, a sudden message from the web or a child who needs attention, or coworkers who require help with their work. These interruptions can drain your focus and cause you to get into the primary task much more challenging.

Zero in on the Smallest Part of Your Work at a Time

One way to kill your mind is to look at your goal as the huge and massive achievement it truly is. Many goals take anywhere from a half-month or more to accomplish and recognizing that may create the impression that taking too much time to think about even thinking about.

It will force you to either:

You are unable to function due to the fact that your goal is big.

Imagine how it will feel to achieve the goal.

Both are detrimental to your focus and always could be a problem when you're focusing into the larger viewpoint or using the sense of.

Everything else being equal, you should center your efforts around doing just a small minimum amount of work.

If, for instance, on the occasion you have to write an article, it's apparent that it will take about 1000 words. If this seems like more than you need, then you should plan to write 200 words each day over the next 5 days (or modify this to meet the requirements at the cut-off date). By separating it into smaller chunks, you makes the entire errand more rational, and assist in determining how avoid getting distracted while on the way.

Picture Yourself Working

In a moment, I mentioned in my tip #4 that the use of representation techniques can hurt the person more than it helps every now and then. There is a method that can be used to legitimately using representation. It's to imagine yourself working.

Champions sprinters employ this method with great success, but generally through working reverse. They visualize themselves as successful at the beginning of their journey before they display the entire race forward, taking in and visualizing every step from the starting point. [1]

The quickest and most effective method of using this technique is to imagine yourself performing just a small portion of the task that needs to be completed.

As an example, in the rare occasion that you're required to rehearse your guitar but you're in the same space (how would we feel about allowing the an extreme amount of sluggishness with this type of model) How would it be advised to handle it?

First imagine standing (truly consider what it would be like to get up, then follow through with the same). If you've really envisioned or imagined it, and you felt the sensation of standing and standing up, at this point, following up with that experience is easy.

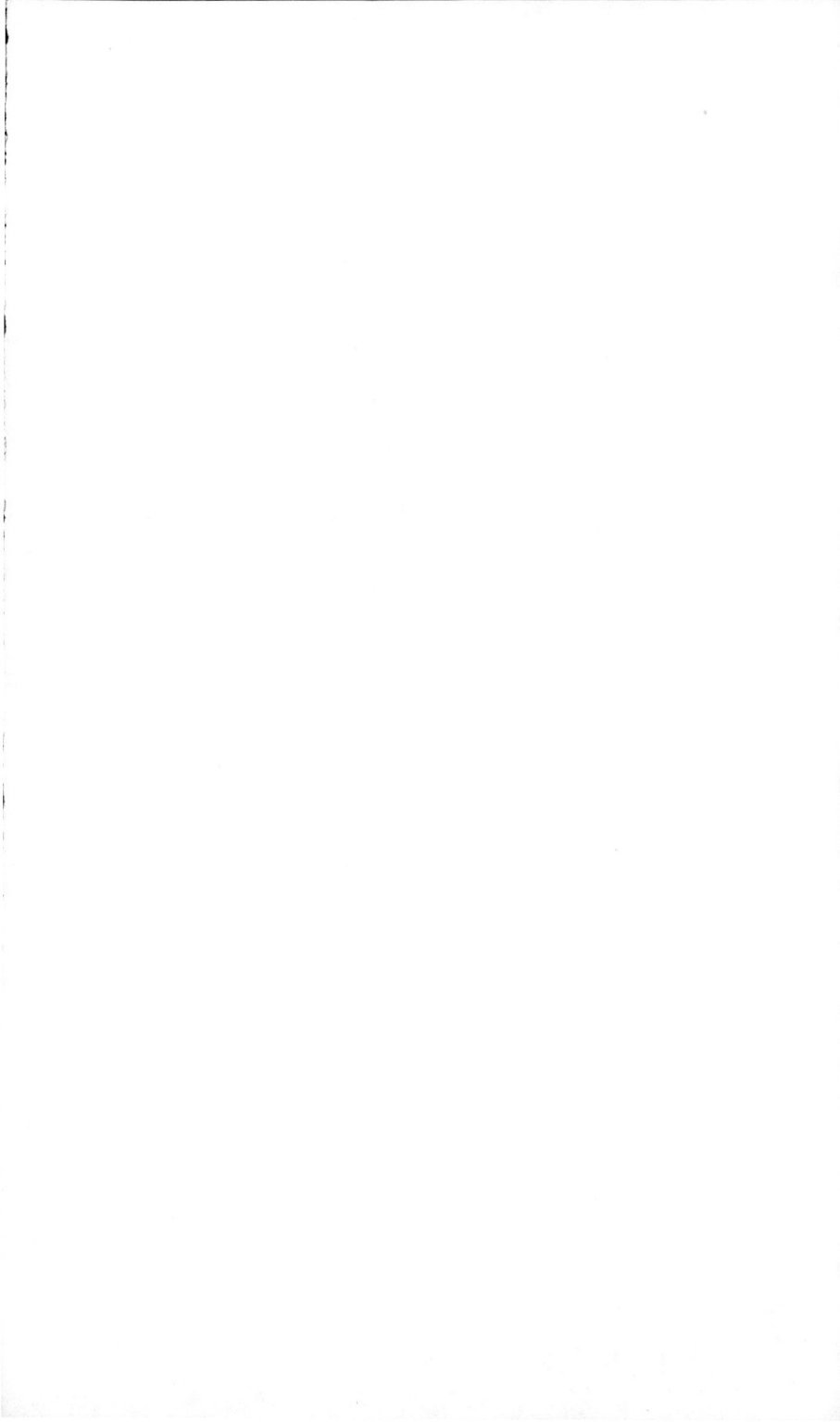